*A Journey
to my Womanhood
Through Endometriosis*

A Journey to my Womanhood Through Endometriosis

MARTA SZYNKIEWICZ

**"To believe in something,
and not to live it, is dishonest."**

—Mahatma Gandhi

I would like to say thank you to the Queens, which have helped me to create this book. Your cheerleading, support and believing in me and my mission was and still is breath taking. Thank you!

Beata Jurasz
Regina Medeiros
Christina Tucciarone
Lenka Jones Photography
Sarah Beaudin
and to all my friends

Dedication

**I dedicate this book to all of the women out
there who want to thrive, and to this pain
and unknown silence in my head,
which I (now) embrace.**

It's been over a year since I first came up with the
idea to write this book. It was a year full of self-doubt,
self-sabotage, and confusion. It consisted of hard
work in order to recover from traumatic surgeries.
It was a year defined by a constant search for ways
to manage my illness. A year to understand that the
'old me', pre-surgery, would not be around anymore,
and I would have to let her go.

 People kept saying to me, "You are strong,"
but somehow I didn't understand what they meant.
Now I do. To go into darkness and fight it all on
your own is the bravest, most magical, and also

the most horrifying thing anybody could ever do. This journey has had the power to break me into a million pieces and to make me whole again so many times over. I'm still going through this process, but now I'm not as scared to fall into pieces anymore. I understand that I'm alive as fuck now!

You may have many people around you, and that's priceless, but they will always perceive you from a certain distance. You will feel their presence, but ultimately, you will be on your own. Any raw experience, any personal transformation requires you to be ALONE.

I'm not here to be your teacher or a guru. I don't claim to have all my shit figured out. All I'm asking is for you to try to touch the feminine strength within you. Don't be afraid to ask questions, and to embrace your power as a WOMAN. You have the entire universe, the biggest library of deep wisdom 'sitting' inside you, just below your belly button — in your womb space.

In a way, experiencing endometriosis has been a spiritual awakening for me.

In this book, I will tell you my story of self-discovery and healing; the raw and honest truth. I will tell you how I grew up and about specific events in my life that have shaped my perception of what being a woman means to me.

On the surface, traumas, sickness, food, and the environments that you live in don't seem to be connected so much. However, during my process of recovery, I have realized that all those components played a crucial role in my healing. I started to understand that my traumas, habits, eating patterns, and much more all had an impact on my health today.

It has been like putting together a huge puzzle representing the bigger picture, yet when you take the pieces apart they make no sense. If you look at them closely one by one, very quickly you will notice that one needs the other to create the whole 'image'. That's the easiest way I can explain how it felt and still feels to explore endometriosis and my place in the world as a woman. This illness was actually a blessing to me. I have learned and discovered so much.

While there is so much to share, this journey is not over. In fact, I've just started.

Foreword

Just before and during the writing of this book, I had lots of resistance and fear. While I consider writing a creative process, it was hard at times to feel like I was fully expressing my feelings.

I had a chat with somebody I met not too long ago and he asked me about how I define creativity and access the feeling of it in my life. Upon reflection, I was quickly able to navigate and find where I was stuck. My most comfortable means of expression is through painting and building. As a set designer, I'm very 'hands on' and I 'talk' through forms, colors, and patterns. Writing, even creative writing, was alien to me as a form of expression.

I started to understand writing as a muscle that I had to stretch and use in order for it to become stronger and more refined. With that realization came a huge sense of relief. I saw that if I put my mind to something and stayed consistent, it could become a reality.

It doesn't matter how other people perceive it... It is YOUR authentic creation, and that's all that matters. With the momentum of practice and possibility, things can only get better.

In this book, I talk about things that might feel unreal or unfamiliar to you. I talk about how I healed and continue to heal myself both in physical and spiritual ways. Now, I can imagine that for some people, physical healing is challenging and at times overwhelming, so spiritual healing might fall lower down on the priority list. Regardless of your point of view, I invite you to start considering healing both aspects of your life congruently. In fact, there is a huge connection between physical healing, mental wellness and the experience of your soul. I invite you to keep an open mind and just jump! Nothing will be the same again.

For my entire life, I felt like I was missing something. There was emptiness in my heart until I became more open, healthy and wealthy. Wealthy with love, awareness, happiness, sadness, and through embracing all life has to offer. I receive it all now! I genuinely feel that we can have everything we ask for and believe in. This book is just a small percentage of what I would love to share with you about this transformation. As I said, I'm stretching when it comes to writing!

I'm typing this chapter on a plane as I return to the UK from France. I'm on the second day of my period. I wouldn't be able to fly and enjoy my life with stage 4 endometriosis and adenomyosis if not for the power of my will, knowledge of manifestation, and a healthy lifestyle. I'm traveling just like a 'normal', 'regular' woman who is on her flow!

Know that it's possible to take back your life and own it fully! Life was given to you to live, to explore, to learn beautiful lessons, to create the life you want, to touch, to laugh, to have amazing sex, to be proud of your achievements, proud of your body, your boobs, your lips! Just look at you! You OWN this and you've got this.

If I can write this book in 6 weeks, imagine what you can do! YOU can do anything you want through belief, a supportive environment, and people who celebrate your health and potential! Eat well, sleep well, set intentions, practice affirmations, dance, move your body, smile, manifest, love yourself, and forgive. I'm with you, closer then you think.

I just looked at my phone to see what song is on because it sounds so beautiful. It's called, "I CARE" by Frances.

Thank you, Universe, and thank you, James, for this beautiful realization around the nature of creating that made this process easier for me.

Contents

CHAPTER ONE

My Story: How I Grew Up

First of all, I would like to say that even if it may seem to you that I'm blaming or pointing to specific events or people as a cause of what I had been through in my life, I don't mean to do that out of anger. I understand that some things just happened and that they played a big part in my healing journey. I believe that all people are fundamentally good but sometimes they lack awareness and understanding towards other human beings. I share these events not to blame, but to paint of picture of how my traumas have informed my journey of sickness and healing.

Before I start, go grab yourself a cup of nice herbal tea or a healthy hot chocolate. My favourite is one made with coconut milk, raw cocoa, maca and coconut butter.

Ready? Let me begin.

I was born in Poland, in a small town called Wabrzezno. I grew up in the village known as Rynsk, on my grandparent's farm.

My childhood was full of contradictions.

I remember having plenty of freedom. I played in the woods, swam in a lake, played with animals and ate fruits straight from a fruit garden. On the other hand, however, I remember my father coming back home drunk, and his aggression towards my sister, my mother and me.

There was constant tension in our house. As a child, you don't really understand what's happening, but you are aware that something isn't right and can sense danger. I didn't understand what feeling secure meant or felt like until I was 30 years old.

I remember one summer evening, my father and my mother were arguing, and he got physical towards her. My mother told me to get my grandparents, and I remember running across the fields to get my nan. If I close my eyes now, I can tell you exactly what the evening light looked like. I still can vividly hear my breath while running and thinking that any minute my father would kill my mother if I didn't run fast enough.

I faced many traumatic events over the years but for some reason this one sticks out in my mind.

I remember the day my father moved out. He hugged me and promised he would be back. He never did. I waited for him for years, never giving up the hope of his return.

Looking back, I can see how much this experience has impacted my relationships; the lack of trust, the pressure to be a good girl, one that deserves for someone to come back to her...

I saw my father once since that day when I went to visit him at his mother's house. I was wearing a dress and he made a comment that my body was too exposed. I was only eight. Later on, as I was falling asleep in the bed we shared, I felt him rubbing up against me.

My body contracted in deep shame and discomfort. I didn't know what exactly was going on but intuitively I knew something wasn't right.

Funny how small events like this one can shape you for life. So small and short-lived, and yet so profound...

This experience definitely 'taught' and conditioned me to feel shame when showing or talking about my body. It was through this incident that I started rejecting my body, and in response, my body weakened and became more vulnerable to illness.

At home we never spoke about feelings. My mother was often sad and anxious. I can see why now. She felt heartbroken and lonely, left to raise two daughters on her own. The word Love was hardly ever used at home.

There was also very little physical interaction. Surviving and feeding us was all my mum could think of at that time. It was almost like we were constantly on alert, never relaxed, and never happy.

Sometimes, unintentionally, she used to tell me that I looked like my father or behaved like him. I knew that he was the reason my mother was sad, so I started to believe that if I was like him, I was also the cause of her sadness.

When I was nine, I started to experience a lot of physical pain. I used to think it was in my tummy. The pain would be so sharp that I would curl up on the ground and couldn't move. I had some medical tests done but some members of my family were convinced that I was making it up. Somehow, the pain just became a part of my life and I stopped talking about it. I thought that's how it should be. I didn't know any different.

Ever since I can remember, I loved creating things whether through building, drawing, writing or painting. It was also my way to cope with the physical and mental pain.

I went to a small primary school in my village. There were only twelve of us in the class, and my teacher Barbara was a loving lady. She used to encourage creativity with us. We made puppets, went on tours to perform, learnt how to play xylophones and created a theatre group. I loved it.

Dear reader, I'm going into so many details here because I want to show you how little events can impact your entire life; how everything happens for a reason and shapes your future. I suggest you stop reading for a moment now and take some time to think about your own childhood. What events and words have stayed in your mind? Sometimes situations that were extremely painful are buried deep inside and you don't even realize they exist. As a child, you decided to put them aside and you forgot they were there, hidden. Maybe you never had anyone to comfort you or to encourage you to look within and face all those uncomfortable feelings. Know that your awareness of these wounds is the first stage of your healing, so I invite you to get curious about what has influenced you up until this point if you are on a journey to wellbeing.

Here are a few more stories of mine.

When I was ten, my mother met a new man. He was a single father of four. Shortly after, we moved into his house and all of a sudden there were six kids living together under one roof.

Neither my sister nor I ever felt quite at home over there. I felt ignored by my mum, who was trying her best to split her attention and energy between all six kids. She had very little room left to experience happiness after going through traumatic years with my father. She also didn't allow herself time to recover before hastily jumping into a new relationship, desperately hoping that it would make her happier.

My mother worked during the day and when she came home after work she would still have so much housework to do that she never had time to talk to me. I'm sure she did her best but as a kid I didn't understand that, and I felt heartbroken.

Sometimes on Saturdays when I wanted to see her, her partner used to lock their bedroom door to prevent me from doing so. She dedicated her entire life to him and his kids. When I wanted to pick her up from work, he used to stop me and send one of his children to pick her up instead. It was incredibly painful.

One afternoon, he brought me downstairs to the basement of our house. Without warning or reason, he made me watch in horror as he strangled my precious pet guinea pig. I never told my mother because I just wanted her to be happy. I knew she would perhaps even dismiss what I told her because she loved him.

Happiness and confidence weren't familiar experiences of mine. Every night I wet my bed until

I was 12. So did my sister. I needed love, but I never felt loved. I'm sure my family was showing me love in their own way, but to me this wasn't enough. It felt like my voice didn't matter.

When I'd started developing into a woman and my body started to change, I remember my breasts hurt so much that I had sleepless nights. I used to walk curled up from pain, so my breasts wouldn't touch my jumper. My mother's partner used to reprimand me for slouching, and when I told him why I couldn't walk straight, he laughed and pinched my breast. Such events in my life have seeded the idea that I should always do what I've been told despite my pain; that I should be ashamed of my changing body; that as a human being, I was insignificant.

My mother had given so much to her partner and his kids, sacrificing her own children as a result. All in vain it seems, because three years later he traded her for a younger woman. We moved out and my mother rented a tiny flat where we stayed for around eight years.

She eventually met another guy, a man who wanted her, but without us, her children. He used to take her out and leave us behind at home. She would go and visit him in Germany where he lived at the time, and every time she came back from those visits, she was angry and took it out on me.

All of this had such a profound impact on my self-perception, my role as a young woman, and my sense of worth. This perception was, and still is, confusing at times. Less now, but the reclaiming of my identity involved a great deal of work.

When I was younger, there was never a "right time" to talk about what or how I felt. I was always mentally tired and in physical pain on a daily basis. Chronic pain affected my ability to solve problems, learn things at school and understand relationships. I passed school and wasn't a bad student, but my memories are foggy. There was nobody to turn to.

When I was thirteen, I got my period for the first time. It was a sunny summer day and I felt so special when I noticed a drop of blood on my knickers. I went to tell my mother and all she said was, "It will go away." She was so casual about it, and I felt deflated and dismissed. Now I realize that her response to it was probably just like the one she had received from her mother, but at that moment I started to associate my period with something that was shameful, inconvenient, taboo, and not worth talking about.

Since that day I started experiencing even more physical discomfort. I can understand the reason now — my endometriosis was progressing, but the time I didn't know. 'Those' days in the month were getting harder to cope with, sometimes forcing me to skip lessons at school from the pain.

The physical pain and lack of understanding around what was going on with my body started to impact my mental health too. I remember feeling sad and lost quite often. I wanted to find answers to how I felt; yet I didn't have any specific questions. I just knew something wasn't right.

After I turned fifteen, I started to look for answers, and for happiness, in men; One after another, the same type of man — the type that wouldn't respect me. To each I would fully submit myself because only then I felt I could be loved. Each of them was 'broken inside' and there I was, so fucking ready to leave everything behind and save them. I would tolerate their abuse and negativity, thinking that if I saved them, I would be their hero, and finally I would be loved.

The truth was, I was broken too, and neither I, nor they benefited from such toxic relationships. I was fulfilling my drive to please people so I could get acceptance from them, and they would abuse me because they didn't love themselves.

Don't get me wrong, it is pleasurable to do nice things for others but only if you also know how to set boundaries. Still to this day I help people, but I do it out of love for myself first. I'm not scared to say NO in fear of someone getting upset with me. If they do, that's their problem! And you should remember that.

At the age of sixteen something happened big enough to nest in my head so profoundly that its impact was irreversible. I was sitting on the sofa of my mother's small flat when she returned home from work with her younger sister, who was coming to visit, and is only 6 years older than me. My mother had bought me a red satin pyjama slip, like a mini dress. It was very cute. I went to try it on, but it was too small for me. After I came back to the room, my mother's sister grabbed it, locked herself in the bathroom and came out saying, "It is good for me, because I'm much slimmer then you." I'm sure she didn't mean for it to hurt, but I was 16 years old and insecure enough already as young woman.

It was at this moment I decided I would lose weight, and that's exactly what happened. In one month, I lost 12 kg. I was so thin. I was eating only 500 kcal per day! I felt so weak and cold all the time and exercised excessively every day. I'd be in my bedroom running in one spot, jumping, doing push ups, etc. Some days I would go for three hours at a time!!! My body was exhausted.

One morning I woke up and fainted from hunger. My mother only then noticed how dangerously skinny I had become. I lost so much hair and my period stopped for over a year. When I went to a doctor because of this problem they said that my womb was abnormal. The doctor told me I may not be able to carry a baby if I didn't stop this drastic diet and put on weight.

But I didn't care. This didn't scare me. Each day I would continue to obsess about what I was going to eat and how many kcal the food had. If I went over my limit, I would extend my exercising time. It was such a mental burden on top of the physical damage I was doing to my body. I see now how little I loved myself. I was slowly killing myself in the name of the short-term fulfilment from losing weight.

It was always never enough. I believed that skinny equalled attractiveness and ultimately, being loveable. On top of that, since my period stopped as a result of such a drastic diet, I experienced less pain in my tummy. This muted the symptoms of my endometriosis, so I was desperate to stay skinny to also keep the pain at bay.

To be fair, to this very day I still haven't managed to make peace with my body, but I feel more relaxed about it now. I love and appreciate my body a lot more. Based on what I went through I can see its beauty and grace. I make sure I do everything I can to support my beautiful temple, but there is still a tiny bit of trauma left deep inside. It's almost like this micro piece of glass stuck in the top of your finger. You can't see it, but once in a while it pinches you to remind you it's still there.

That's all I want to tell you about my childhood and growing up. I'm sure I missed some things, but the main events are out there for you to read, to get to know me and to provoke you, my dear reader, to get to know yourself better. It is crucial in your journey of self-healing to develop a loving relationship with your body and the messages it is sending you.

Just like me, you might have experienced some ignorance and lack of awareness when you tried to talk about your pain with others. This is why this reflection process is so important, so that you learn how to trust yourself and what you feel, but also so that you realize you have to heal both your heart, soul AND your body to experience holistic fulfilment.

CHAPTER TWO

Endo, Adeno... What?

I'm sure you have already done some research on what endometriosis and adenomyosis are before you've even opened this book. When I experienced a bleeding colon three years ago and started searching Google for answers, the word *Endometriosis* was one of the main links that popped out in the search bar. However, all the main websites contained exactly the same information, as if they had copied and pasted from one source.

I eventually realized that most of the information had contained myths, but for a long time, I experienced a lot of worry around the condition. I wish that back then I'd had access to other, more personal types of information on those illnesses, stories that were written by women who had actually experienced endometriosis. There really is very little accurate information out there, and that's the main reason I decided to write this book.

Remembering this just makes me realize how much work I have done on my own to get to the other side and become stronger. I am walking proof that YOU CAN live a relatively pain-free life with endometriosis if you're determined to do so. You can have a dream job, play sports, and travel. I would even go as far as to say that experiencing endometriosis could benefit your life in that it can make you stronger, more resilient. I know that if you are going through this illness and reading this book you might now wish to close it and throw it in my face. And I don't blame you. But bear with me.

Writing this chapter has proven to be the most challenging compared to all other chapters in my book. This is because in order to write about it, I had to try and go back to emotions and feelings that I experienced three years ago when I realized that there was definitely something wrong with my body. I wanted to remember how this alien feeling felt, having something that was literally breaking open inside of me.

Let me start from the beginning with what Endometriosis and Adenomyosis actually are. I will try to explain it in as simple terms as possible. A woman has a womb/uterus, an organ that was designed by the universe for her to carry a baby. The womb contains cells that are called *Endometrium Cells*. Endometrium cells are responsible for providing the lining of the womb, and become thicker each month, preparing for potential conception. If conception doesn't happen, endometrium cells shed, which is referred to as menstruation, or more commonly, a period. Now if a woman experiences endometriosis, her endometrium cells travel in other directions. Instead of going *with the flow* and exiting through the vagina, they travel the opposite way through the fallopian tubes and either camp out in the fallopian tubes, the ovaries, or in the spaces around your abdomen. They sit on the walls of a woman's organs. They can even travel as far as to the brain! But this is rare. The most popular places in which they often stay are the bladder, kidney, colon, ovaries, fallopian tubes, stomach, the walls of the woman's belly, or the walls of the womb.

Adenomyosis is a manifestation of endometriosis where endometrium cells grow into and get 'stuck' inside the walls of the womb. With time, they are likely to form tumors or lumps. Unfortunately, it is impossible to remove adenomyosis without removing the entire womb.

After these endometrium cells find their spot to 'settle', they react exactly like the normal endometrium cells in your womb. So each time you have a period, endometrium cells in your abdomen or in affected organs (yes, endo cells can go deep into an organ's wall and get inside them) bleed as they would in the womb. Unfortunately, the blood of endometrium cells can escape and go anywhere in the body, forming lesions and scar tissue that grow with each menstruation cycle.

Some lesions get stuck to one another, which in turn can paralyze organs, merge them together or even relocate them. This all contributes to the pain that each person experiences with the illness. On top of that, your immune system does not understand that those cells actually belong to your body. It thinks they are foreign cells. The immune system then becomes alert and starts to fight them. It's a very complicated and intense process that puts you in a high state of inflammation. Just think about it! Every month your body gets full of bleeding cells that are unable to escape! It's a constant struggle.

Also, if you have endometrium cells on ovaries, quite often you can experience cysts called chocolate cysts. They are called this because they are full of old blood, which has a chocolaty color. I had one of them myself, and it popped just after the bleeding started in my colon. A breaking of chocolate cysts can be extremely dangerous, so if you are an *endo girl*, make sure you have your ovaries checked on a regular basis for any cysts.

Ok, so that's the endometriosis explained objectively. Now, I would like to talk about some information that you may come across in your own research to which I strongly disagree. Hence, I refer to it as myths. It is important to say that I am not a doctor so I can only speak from my own experience and that of other women with endometriosis whom I interviewed for this book.

Myth 1: **Hysterectomy is a cure for endometriosis.**

Such nonsense! Having your uterus removed doesn't mean your endometriosis will stop. Let me explain this to you in a very simple way. Imagine you have endometriosis and a doctor wants to remove your uterus. There are two options for doing so:

The first is to remove only the womb and the second is to remove both the ovaries and the womb. For now, let's talk about the first option. The womb has been removed, but you might still have some endometrium cells left behind by your doctor. Your ovaries are still 'working' and stimulating all their hormones just like they do. Those endometrium cells left behind will continue to grow and bleed in response to your natural hormones, which your ovaries still produce.

Why am I so convinced a doctor would leave some cells behind during a hysterectomy? The majority of doctors will only remove some scar tissue and lesions. They will not shave each organ to remove the potential microcells. The majority of doctors are not that skilled. Even for skilled doctors, it's challenging to remove everything.

The same issues apply when you have both the womb and ovaries removed. If the ovaries are removed, then chances are you will have to take a hormone replacement, which carries an inherent risk of increasing the recurrence of the illness. Endometrium cells cannot recognize if the hormones present are natural or synthetic. The cells will respond the same and continue to bleed. In my opinion, doctors suggest to opt for hysterectomies in these situations way too often.

Myth 2: **If you are at Stage 1 of the condition, meaning that there's not a lot of overgrowth of the endometrium cells, you have less pain than Stage 4 growth.**

This is not always the case. Research has shown that 20% of women experiencing endometriosis at Stage 1 or 2 can have the exact same symptoms as women with Stage 3 or 4. The intensity of those symptoms can be just as high. It all depends on which organs are involved and in which places the lesions and scar tissues form.

Myth 3: **Endometriosis is a chronic illness and therefore, nothing but a hysterectomy and heavy drugs can help you.**

Well, this is where I will step in with personal experience. Over 10 doctors have told me in recent years that I should have a hysterectomy and go under hormone replacement therapy. Instead, I dove into intense research and plenty of tests and experiments to prove that a woman with endometriosis and adenomyosis can improve the quality of her life while keeping her womb and ovaries intact and functioning. It involves a lot of hard work but it's possible. The right diet, supplements, tests, and relaxation techniques can all help tackle your pain and improve the quality of your life.

Myth 4: **It's normal to be prescribed certain drugs without being properly diagnosed first.**

How can you treat something you didn't even see or know much about? Every woman who potentially has endometriosis should be diagnosed via laparoscopy first, which is a surgery that allows you to view the organs in the abdomen before any prescription drugs are given.

Prescription drugs can have lots of side effects, especially the ones that aim to put you into the state of menopause. Unfortunately, doctors often fail to inform the women about all the side effects.

If you decide to take the route of using prescription drugs, make sure that you are efficiently tested and diagnosed first, and inform yourself on the side effects of any medication.

Myth 5: **It's just a heavy period.**

I remember going from doctor to doctor and hearing "It's just a heavy period" countless times. I've also been told that my pain was "only in my head" or to "stop being a woman about it." It's very painful to be dismissed like that when you're searching for help. In fact, such responses can even discourage you from seeking help. But I assure you; it is not only in your head!

Experiencing endometriosis has really made me tune into my body and become more aware of its needs. It's hard to believe but the pain and the sensations you feel can be a powerful opportunity for transformation. It might not be so clear to you just yet but if you put in some work to see the gift, just like I did and continue to do, magic will unfold. Experiencing your period does not have to be associated with unbearable pain.

Myth 6: **Pregnancy is a cure for endometriosis.**

I am full of mixed emotions about this one. It is hard to comprehend that in this day and age some doctors will still look for such 'short cuts' knowing full well that pregnancy DOES NOT cure endometriosis, just pauses it temporarily. It makes me sad thinking that some women will fall for it, desperate for the pain to end. They decide to have a child out of fear and not love.

Myth 7: **Women with endometriosis suffer pain only during their menstruation.**

Any of you who have experienced endometriosis will know only too well that this statement is far from the truth. For me, the first half of the cycle is relatively pain-free, but the second part tends to be extremely painful and uncomfortable. My tummy gets tender and swollen. A couple of days before my period I often feel like I'm already bleeding. On top of that, sudden flare-ups can come and go out of the blue, lasting anywhere from a couple of minutes to hours, or even days. There is no pattern to describe the type of pain I experience each month. It is all rather unpredictable.

Myth 8: **You can only experience endometriosis when you start your ovulation.**

That's not true. Girls can suffer from endometriosis pain even before they experience their first menstrual cycle due to pre-menstrual hormone changes.

Myth 9: **Endometriosis can be caused by infections such as STDs, and can be cured with antibiotics.**

I think the main problem here is mixing up the spelling of two very similar words: endometriosis and endometritis. Endometritis is an inflammation of the inner lining of the uterus and can be caused by sexually transmitted diseases or even tuberculosis. Just like with everything I have shared with you, I invite you to do your own research. I never take any information for granted, even if it comes from the medical experts. I always question all statements and look for my own answers. It doesn't mean I don't trust the doctors, it just means I value my own research and experience.

"The important thing is to not stop questioning."

—Albert Einstein

CHAPTER THREE

Diagnosis & Surgery

Before I sat down to write this chapter I was worried that I wouldn't be able to trace the exact moment I started to feel unwell. To my surprise, I didn't have that problem at all. The memory came back vividly.

When you're young and growing up on a farm, you get used to pain, be it from climbing trees or falling over while running and exploring. Around ten years old, something changed. I was playing outside in the summer and suddenly got such strong cramps in my abdomen that I had to lie down on the ground. I stayed curled up in a ball until the intensity subsided. It was confusing, different then other pain I'd experienced. However, I dismissed it, not realizing how abnormal it actually was. I didn't know it at the time, but this was when I first started suffering from endometriosis. It all makes sense now.

As the years went on, the pain became more frequent and intense, coming and going like waves. Since beginning ovulation at thirteen, I never knew anything other than painful periods. I remember the pain being so bad at times that I couldn't leave my bed. It was excruciating. The bleeding got so heavy that there was always an embarrassing patch of blood on my trousers. No amount of pads would help.

My back and legs would swell, making it hard to walk or bend over. Still, I forced myself to go to school and even attend exercise lessons. I'd also experience sweats, fevers, headaches, and double vision. Sometimes, even touching any part of my body would generate discomfort. Urination was painful and bowel movements, even more so. Blood would often leak out of my colon. More often than not I was dizzy, bloated and extremely tired. Mood swings and anxiety attacks were common. Certain foods also made me sick, but I'll talk more about that in another chapter.

The pain continued to increase in my late twenties and by the time I was in my thirties I had to plan my life around my cycle. Despite how challenging this was, I never questioned the pain. I thought that it was normal, whatever normal means, and I didn't talk about it since it felt taboo to even have a period.

During the writing of this chapter, I started to look for notes, pictures or videos that I recorded during these flare-ups. I came across a terrifying video of me crying at 2am, having recorded my experience after a third sleepless night and two visits to the emergency room. Each time, the hospital sent me home with just painkillers. On the screen, my face was red and my eyes, so swollen you could hardly see them. I was begging for answers and for somebody to help me, desperate and to some degree, without hope.

I cried looking back at this video while simultaneously realizing the beauty of that moment. Reflecting on it now, I'm reminded of why I'm writing this book. I'm writing it for YOU and sharing this powerful memory so that you know I understand the depths of pain endometriosis can trigger.

The night of that video I had also been researching for a private hospital to have a hysterectomy. I was so protective over my womb and ovaries but in that moment of suffering, I was looking for any relief. While I didn't go through with it, mentally I felt prepared, and for me, it felt as though I had already done it.

I also admire women who decide to have a hysterectomy. Please know you are not any less just because you don't have a womb or ovaries. You still have space, a magical space where the energy of your womb and ovaries is still present. You get to honor this space with all your heart and soul.

While this memory of sleepless suffering was intense enough, the biggest wakeup call for me was an accident that happened during sex. I had a cyst growing on my left ovary that I wasn't aware of, and during intercourse, it popped. It felt like all my organs were about to fail. My heart began to race and thought I was going to have diarrhea, vomit, and pee myself. Burning, sharp waves of pain rippled from my neck to my anus.

I immediately went to the hospital. After a short inspection, they let me out without thoroughly investigating what would have caused the cyst to grow in the first place. My body had to continue dealing with it on its own. Body bless you! I love you!

Days passed and the pain got more and more intense. I got weaker and weaker each month and year. It was difficult to perform simple functions. Even lifting a cup with tea was a challenge at times.

I lied about my symptoms a lot. It was just so tricky to explain how I felt, and often it felt in vain, especially when doctors started to suggest it was "all in my head." Sometimes I prayed for something to take me and end it all.

Each doctor I saw would tell me something different. I'd hear everything from, "That's just womanhood… a normal period" to, "It's in your head" or, "You need to see a psychologist." It was a very lonely place to be, the land of the misunderstood. At some point, I started to believe them and question myself, thinking I was going crazy. I tried to dismiss what I was really feeling, slowly drowning in a sad, lonely place.

During the last four years, I saw over ten different doctors before my pain became absolutely unbearable. In 2016, I noticed more bleeding from my colon, but not like in the past. It wasn't just drops. This time it was a flow of blood. I went to my doctor at the time to share this scary discovery, and his reaction shocked me. After administering zero tests, he sent me home with a packet of painkillers stating, "It's definitely a hemorrhoid."

I remember this wave of hopelessness moving over me. Sitting on the bench in front of his office, I watched people passing by, feeling so empty, lonely and lost. Back home, I pulled down my pants and stared at the red patch on my underwear, fresh blood from my colon.

It took me a few days to get myself together and understand that I had to take further action to protect myself. I also realized I had two choices; lie down and believe I'd never live a normal life, or take things into my own hands and fight for my health with all I had left. That's when I started researching my symptoms.

During my research, the word 'endometriosis' kept showing up. I remember it like yesterday, finding a list of symptoms on an endometriosis charity website, and checking each of them off. A hot wave of fear passed through me as I read that I am a "1 in 10" statistic of women suffering from this condition! How? Why? In those moments I was filled with confusion and resistance.

During my research, I also found out that one way to try and get rid of endometriosis is to have a full hysterectomy, and even then some women still experience pain. There's no guarantee it would help. It's a gamble that women have to take full responsibility for, and I didn't want to go this route. I was 32 years old and desired kids, joyful sex, and the ability to dance, travel and do sports. But back then I was barely able to get myself to university and home. I wasn't living… I was just surviving.

I went to my local doctor with the print outs from different websites I'd researched and demanded to see a specialist. I had to go FIVE times before they referred me to a gynecology clinic, which took four months to get into! During this time I continued doing my own research. My life was consumed with learning as much as I could about this illness. I quickly understood that I had to be willing to become friends with her and get to know her as much as I could. I had to live with her 24/7, 365 days a year, probably for the rest of my life.

When the date of my appointment finally arrived, I made my way to the hospital with a file FULL of research pages and e-mails from other doctors and women who had experience with endometriosis. To my surprise (again!), he knew maybe 30% of what I did! It felt like being in a bad dream. I did receive some empathy and the proposal of a hysterectomy or laser surgery, which is so not effective. It was another disappointment, and more hours spent crying on a bench outside of the hospital.

When I got back home, I remember touching my tummy and begging, "Please, show me the way." The very next day I found an amazing doctor who specialized only in endometriosis, had amazing patient results and didn't believe in short cuts. He had his own private hospital and was very well known. I booked an appointment immediately for two months out, despite the high expense. I knew I needed to see him.

Those two months felt like forever. Each day my pains were getting worse. Sometimes I was brought to my knees in the middle of the street, on trains or in shops. The pain would come unexpected, unexplained.

My appointment finally arrived, and by then I had doubled the size of the file I brought with me. The doctor was very direct and I felt like I was FINALLY speaking with someone who 'gets it'. He told me I also have adenomyosis (endo cells growing inside the walls of my womb). He also said that based on the years of my suffering, the intensity of pain, and the organs involved I'd most likely be at stage 4 of the condition, the most invasive level. He talked about surgery options and the pros and cons. While it was a relief to finally have some answers, I was also devastated. I had known I was sick but I didn't realize how bad it was, or the risk and damage that endometriosis could do to my organs.

We scheduled a date for my first diagnostic surgery. It was another two months away, giving me some time to figure out how I would pay for it. I knew I had to remain with this doctor. A regular gynecologist wouldn't be able to perform surgery on an illness that could be in your bladder, colon, kidney, or other organs. They're not qualified enough to do that and while a hysterectomy is toted as a "cure", it's an inefficient short cut, a price we women with endo pay for lack of education.

During preparation for my surgery, I was completing my Masters degree and my finals were just a couple of days before the surgery date. My anticipation to finally find out more around my condition gave me the strength to finish strong. I passed my exams with amazing grades. I didn't have much time or will to celebrate so in the days before surgery I stayed in bed, recovering from mental exhaustion.

On the 15th of September 2016, I had my diagnosis surgery. It took seven hours. The doctor worked to separate all of my organs from each other, as they were enmeshed due to the lesions and dead scar tissue. Some of my organs had been relocated for years and were deformed. It all looked like a big cocoon.

When I woke up from the general anesthetic, the doctor gave me the diagnosis — Aggressive Stage 4, Recto-vaginal, meaning that it was affecting over four organs and my colon was fused to my womb.

Of the organs affected were my bladder, colon, kidney, fallopian tubes, ovaries, stomach, and womb. He said it was one of the worst cases he'd ever come across in 25 years of treating endometriosis.

A second surgery for Radical Endometriosis Excision was scheduled for three months out. This is a procedure where the doctor removes old endometrium lesions and scar tissue through very delicate incisions. It's a specialist/niche surgery that requires extensive training and precision to be done effectively. He said that the operating time could take anywhere from ten to fourteen hours. He also informed me about the risks involved when operating on so many organs at once. There was a big possibility of damaging organs. I was so afraid but KNEW I had to give it a chance.

Those next three months were very lonely and sad. Nobody really knew how to give me support, including myself. When people have cancer at least you can see they are sick. However, I looked healthy on the outside so I struggled to ask for support because I felt like no one would truly understand. Either way, I couldn't fully prepare mentally and physically for what was about to come.

January 6th, 2017: The day I went in for my Radical Endometriosis Excision. Even writing about it now, after two years have passed, I can still remember how afraid I was. It was one of the scariest days of my life. Petrified is the only word I can think of that describes it accurately. I'm crying now thinking about it.

We arrived at the hospital the day before for blood tests and pre-surgery consultation. I don't remember exactly what the doctor told me that day. Everything was and still is foggy when I think back.

The next day I checked in to the hospital at 6:30 am. My surgery was scheduled for 7:30 am. Just before going in I was given a long list of papers to sign regarding the potential risks. It felt pointless. I had no choice but to have this surgery, to give my organs a fighting chance. I was neglected for too long by other doctors and by ME for not owning my voice. I had to do this and take back my power.

As I walked in, my legs felt wobbly and weak. I turned to say goodbye to my friend Daria who was there with me. Her smile is one of the only things I remember well from that day. It felt unreal to be there.

I was put on a bed and told that as soon as I fell asleep, they would move me to a special 'star' bed shaped like an X. This was so that when the doctors stripped my ligaments they could rotate me in order to access all my organs. I was also told I might have very swollen arms, legs, and head, as I would be hanging upside down during surgery. The last thing I said to my doctor before going under was, "Please save me."

Twelve hours later, a wave of vomit woke me up. There were many people pulling at my legs and arms. I couldn't open my eyes or move my head. I continued to vomit. Behind my eyelids, I saw vibrating white dots and felt extreme pain in my feet and hands. I felt someone putting more drugs into the IV in my hand.

After an hour or so they moved me into my room. I still couldn't open my eyes. All I heard was my own heavy breathing and felt a pain in my feet that was unbearable. I wanted to die. In fact, I thought that's what was happening for a little while. By 3 am they came to remove some tubes and the catheter. Sleeping felt impossible.

By the morning, the pain started to ease up. At around 8 am, two nurses came and tried to persuade me to use the toilet. I was so pained and swollen it was difficult for me to even respond. I didn't feel ready but they helped to lift me off the bed and sit me on a chair. I almost fainted twice. I managed to pee a bit and begged them to put me back in bed.

I spent the day after my surgery in post-traumatic shock. I still wasn't able to open my eyes, this time not from a swollen face. I just didn't have the energy. My heart rate was very high and I trembled and sweat. I felt cold on the outside and hot on the inside. It's impossible to fully describe what I felt, and I never expected that my body could handle so much.

I spent four days at the hospital and an extra night at a hotel nearby. Because of the distance to drive back home, the doctors requested I stay close, just in case of unexpected complications. On the second day post-surgery I started to feel more responsive, and with the help of my friend, I managed to wash myself sitting down. My hands, feet, and head were still so swollen. My feet were so big and round I hardly could walk. Every step was painful. I had so many bruises on my body from the belts and the bed I was operated on. Later on, I found out I had hung upside down for over seven out of the twelve hours in surgery.

During the excision, they separated and shaved the top layer of tissue from seven organs to make sure they had removed every possible endometrium cell. Upon finishing, they had filled my belly with a special liquid so my organs could heal without sticking to one another. My belly felt like a huge balloon and I easily looked nine months pregnant. On top of that, I had my ovaries stitched up against the walls of my belly, so they wouldn't stick to any of my healing organs. I had them suspended for ten whole days.

Leaving the hospital, I cried hysterically all the way to the car. It felt like a huge release of energy that had been stuck in my body for so long. It was also in response to the relief I felt around surviving the surgery, the remaining physical pain, and a feeling that my body had been violated. I know my doctor had just saved me but I also had this feeling like I'd been abused. I felt very vulnerable and emotional.

Like I said before, nothing and nobody could have ever prepared me for what had happened and what was about to happen. From then on, every step, every word, move, walk, and every meal was a small victory.

Notes from my journal post-surgery:

"It's time. It's time to heal. It's time to say goodbye to you, cells. I'm sorry that you had to leave my body. I love you. You were like my little babies. You were a part of me. My heart is racing and I can't focus. It's going to be ok. Thank you."

CHAPTER FOUR

Recovery

Recovery wasn't easy. After coming home, I stayed in bed the entire first week, barely moving. My friend came over twice a day to help me shower, make me a big flask of tea, bring me food, and help me change. I didn't sleep much because the pain was so insidious. When I'd shift my body, I could feel my organs rubbing up against each other. It was quite strange and unsettling. That first week dragged on.

Eventually, the swelling started to come down, and I could fully open my eyes and move my feet. The bruising on my body started to change from dark blue to yellow. I felt a bit better but still looked like the victim of a violent accident.

Going to the toilet was the most challenging for me. My bladder, colon, and kidney were the organs most affected by the endometriosis, so it was very painful for me to wee or poo. The doctor did warn me that while he did all he could to remove as much dead scar tissue and lesions as possible, he wasn't able to guarantee full recovery of my organs.

Eventually though, the pain did go away. I remember sitting on the toilet and thinking, "What a big blessing it is to just have a 'normal' wee." I never expected I could be so grateful for every pain-free drop of urine!

The second week was slightly easier. My bruising and swelling continued to improve. The pain also became easier to handle. I'm not sure if this was because I just got used to it, or if it actually started to lessen.

My ovary suspension was scheduled for removal by the end of that week. I was very scared because I knew it would be uncomfortable. The strings holding my ovaries against the wall of my stomach had to be threaded out *through* my stomach wall, and I wasn't looking forward to another invasive procedure.

When the time came, I was fully awake without painkillers. Normally it's not unbearable, but right away there was a small complication. One of the strings didn't want to move. It was either tangled around my ovaries or stuck in a blood clot. The doctor struggled to pull it out, wiggling it around in different directions with more force than usual. It was very painful, and I prayed for it to release so that I didn't have to go under again.

Finally, it came loose, and I felt my ovaries drop back into place inside my belly. The sensation was surreal. For the first time in what felt like forever, I recognized what it was like to really connect to my body.

As each week passed, I felt better and better. Every day I discovered that I could stretch my independence a little further. Things people take for granted like putting on shoes, bending over, and making tea became small celebrations. It took me about two months to get to the point where I could walk my dog and do small activities like drive my car, go food shopping, and do some housework. Even then I wasn't fully recovered.

I'd been told that a full recovery could take about a year, and even then my pain would not fully subside. Along the way, there were days when I'd have no pain, followed by days where it felt as though the pain was making up for lost time. Nothing was certain. Everything was fragile.

With all the unpredictability, sometimes I'd still question if it was worth fighting for. Each month, my periods were different. You would think by then I would have given up observing and staying curious about my body, but I knew I had to keep checking in. The sensations in my body wouldn't allow me to avoid and ignore it the way I used to. My relationship with them was different. I was learning about myself all over again.

In the months to follow, I would wake up in the middle of the night, crying and disoriented, flashing back to the days just before and after the procedure. My emotions in the wake of recovery were like a roller coaster. Physically I felt weak, but at the same time, extremely strong and proud of what I was able to survive and move through.

During this time I didn't have sex, even when my doctor told me that it would be fine. I was single anyway but also scared that intercourse would do further damage and complicate recovery. My sole focus was on healing and loving myself again. Every day was about cooking the right things, wearing the right things, and planning my movements. A partner was the last thing on my mind.

The surgery wasn't a complete cure. At the end of the first year, my colon was still bleeding during my period. Unfortunately, it was so damaged by the endometriosis that the doctor wasn't able to remove all the endometrium cells. There was too much of a risk that my colon would become permanently damaged. He'd left some scar tissue behind hoping it would die naturally, but that wasn't the case. It grew back. I also continued to experience 'full bladder' sensations and painful urination on occasion.

However, my periods improved overall. Before surgery, I'd stay in bed for the entirety of the bleeding, up to five days at a time. A year post-surgery, I was able to leave the house just a few days after my bleeding started. I stopped lying to people about my symptoms and became more mobile. The pain in my joints and back was less noticeable and I could accomplish all my daily tasks without suffering. In general, I saw about a 50% improvement of symptoms, and for someone who wasn't able to even make herself a cup of tea when on her period, this shift felt like a miracle.

The surgery was and still is one of my biggest traumas and teachers. In the beginning, I had hoped that it would fix me. What I learned is that instead, it was the jumpstart I needed to take my power back and stand up for myself. I learned that I had to be my own healer, friend, doctor, and supporter, that it was up to me to maintain this 50% increase in freedom that my doctor gave me and to continue the recovery process with integrity and determination.

It sounds exhausting, and yes, sometimes it was. But this commitment has become an integral part of who I am. In fact, my recovery routine is the most solid part of my life. It's my security blanket, the only thing that I can take control of. It's so normal for me to live comfortably with endometriosis now. Deep down inside, I knew all along that with time, I could heal myself, and you can too.

CHAPTER FIVE

How to Live with Endometriosis and Maintain a Pain-Free Life

I'm about to share the lifestyle shifts that helped speed up my recovery and now allow me to live comfortably with endometriosis. I'm not a doctor, and the information I share is based on my own extensive research, personal experience, and the experience of other women with endometriosis whom I connected with along my journey. My research is solid, yet it's still just mine, and I can't promise that all of it will help you find relief. I invite you to try on anything that resonates and to check in with YOUR body to see what feels good for you.

I know one thing for sure: an open mind, a spark of hope, the will to commit, and a system of consistent, effective routines will bring positive results.

Let me start with my core belief, which is:

ENDOMETRIOSIS IS NOT A RANDOM ILLNESS. IT IS A RESULT OF AN IMBALANCED IMMUNE SYSTEM.

Maybe this is new to you. Maybe it sounds nuts. But know that endometriosis, just like many other illnesses, is a side effect of a much bigger issue.

Our bodies have the capability to recover pretty much from anything. Organically, our precious bodies want to live, to serve us, to thrive. But when a person's immune system does not have a healthy environment to nurture it, when it's fed toxins and stress day in and day out, it starts to act up. Once you have this awareness, no matter what's happened in your past, it becomes your responsibility to decide what kind of an environment you want to create for it in the present.

As soon as I started seeing my body as an organism that is always fighting for me, I knew that I had to meet it halfway, to become a warrior for my army of cells, to love it into repair. The list of tools, resources, and practices I'm sharing with you below are the result of this conviction. I invite you to get curious about this offering. Take notes, do your own research, and invite in the possibility that you too have the power to heal. In the back of the book, I will provide a list of the most helpful resources that I used along the way so that you can start somewhere too.

ORGANIC FOOD

"Let food be thy medicine and medicine be thy food."
—*Hippocrates*

In today's world, so much of consumption marketing focuses on "the best deals" and "saving money." As a consequence, we settle for genetically modified and processed foods. I refer to them as "fake grown foods" because it's not natural for vegetables and fruits to grow "as fast as possible" and end up being "perfect," void of bugs or dirt. The number of pesticides and chemicals used to grow fruits and veggies is terrifying, and that's not even taking into consideration the chemicals added to packaged foods.

Unfortunately, the consequences of consuming these chemicals are not widely shared, but research has connected excessive consumption of modified and processed foods to many adverse health conditions. Just some of the side-affects measured include nausea, vomiting, stomach problem, headaches, dizziness, weakness, confusion, chest pains, body aches, heart problems, cancer, and other chronic illnesses.

Eating organic has had a HUGE impact on my ability to recover from surgery and improve my health. I started eating organic about five years ago in 2013. That was even before I diagnosed myself with endometriosis. My awareness shifted after a friend of mine told me that she cured her child of some skin condition just through changing his diet. The doctors told her that he'd never be able to tolerate sun exposure, but the boy is twelve years old now and sunbathes every summer! Naturally, it piqued my curiosity.

I started slow, by making sure that at least my leafy greens and veggies were organic, like spinach, lettuce, cucumbers, etc. Then as I got used to that I began to buy organic food across the board. Right away I noticed that I had more energy and less brain fog, and over time, my skin cleared up, my hair got stronger and the white of my eyes got brighter.

I also found that with a bit of research and effort, it's possible to eat healthy, even on a small budget. Local markets and most grocery stores now have an organic section, and while the cost is a bit more, I'd rather pay more now than suffer the medical costs later for the health issues caused by chemicals. Also, I noticed that the more I paid for food, the more appreciative of it I became. I waste much, much less than I used to when the food felt more disposable.

Looking back, I'm amazed that I didn't recognize the food/health connection earlier. I was ignorant, but I know now that I fell prey to the marketing of misinformation that permeates society. In many ways, we're being brainwashed to eat poison. No wonder why there are so many diseases. I don't want to push you into the land of fear, because that's not the point. What I want is to invite you to take ownership of what you are putting into your body and recognize that your food choices determine how you feel.

For me, there is no compromising on food. I see this as a logical situation. I eat healthily; therefore I can work, travel, earn money, enjoy my life, write this book, walk my dogs, drive, see friends and family, and live a full life. When I don't eat healthily, I become unwell and can't do anything. The math is simple!

As I said, this beautiful organism is designed to recover from pretty much every illness if you give it the right environment and foods. Food is medicine — it's as simple as that. Even the greatest minds of our time knew that. You are what you eat, so if you want to feel healthy and alive, make sure that the food you eat is organic and alive.

TYPES OF FOOD I AVOID

It took me a lot of time, testing, and observing to figure out which foods serve my body and which ones don't. Through conversing with other women who were also experiencing endometriosis, I found that the foods that irritated me also irritated them. I also found studies showing that some foods cause inflammation in most bodies, and definitely should be avoided, especially by women with endometriosis.

My proposition to you is to start your own journal where you log everything you eat each day, and how it makes you feel. Note any pain, flare-ups, or other changes. It will take some effort and time, but it will pay off, I promise.

Here is my personal "AVOID" list:

- **Processed food** — Essentially any food that has been altered in some ways during preparation. This is the majority of the foods in supermarkets. Some examples are breakfast cereals, biscuits, canned vegetables, sausages, ham, cheese, ready-made microwave meals, pastries, crisps, etc.

- **Wheat** — Wheat may potentially lead to inflammation in the lymph nodes, kidneys, spleen, and brain. Avoiding wheat is not the same as avoiding gluten. Gluten is a mixture of two proteins that are added to food or even to cosmetics to keep things together. I avoid gluten too, but not as religiously as wheat.
- **Refined sugar** — I don't think I have to say a lot about sugar. Most know how harmful sugar is for the body. It can cause diabetes, weight gain, problems with your hearing, and increases the chance of getting cancer (sugar feeds cancer cells!). I still eat sweet things in moderation, but when I do I make sure they have agave, honey, date syrup, coconut sugar, cane sugar, or xylitol instead of refined sugar.
- **Dairy** — I dropped milk from my diet over five years ago and cheese two years ago. To start with, it was only because I felt sorry for animals. With time I discovered many other side effects that milk and its by-products have on our body. Antibiotics and hormones are pumped into farmed cows, and small amounts of pus get into distributed milk due to the cows being so unhealthy. All of that can have a big impact on your own health, most often

increasing inflammation in the body. The best alternatives to regular cheese or milk are nut-based products, which are readily available at groceries stores now. If you are allergic to nuts you can get oat milk.

- **Soy** — I'm avoiding at all cost because it's a GMO (genetically modified organism), which basically mean its human-made food. To me, it's not natural and doesn't feel right to eat.
- **Nightshade vegetables** — These are on my 'sometimes' list. I'm trying my best to avoid them, but I'll eat them on occasion if they're in a dish that I fancy. Some examples of nightshades are tomatoes, potatoes, aubergine, and peppers.

WATER

"Water and our necessary food are the only things that wise men must fight for."

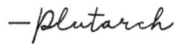

—*Plutarch*

The quote sounds simple, I know, but our body is made up of 55-65% of water! That's right. More than half of you is made up of water. When I found this out during my recovery, I started to look into how much water I consumed and the quality of that water. I spent a week reading books from doctors, researchers, and holistic gurus just to learn as much as I could. I went through many kinds of filters for my water and tested it often at a lab to find out what chemicals were inside and how toxic it might be.

In this short chapter, I will share only a bit of what I've learned. It's a 'deep water' subject, so I encourage you to continue doing your own research.

Generally speaking, tap water is very harmful to us. It contains up-cycled antibiotics, fluoride, chlorine, and pesticides. Harmful effects of chlorine are increased risk of cancer, cell damage, increased risk of asthma, and heart problems, to name a few. Fluoride can lead to bone disease and problems with your thyroid.

After finding out how dangerous tap water can be, I thought that bottled water was the way to go, but very quickly I found out that 50% of bottle water still contains the same chemicals as tap water! Even worse, it contains one more chemical, which when it comes to women's health is a killer — Dioxin. Dioxin is in the plastic, and it's a fake hormone. It acts like a hormone in our body but our bodies can't recognize it. Once inside our system, it complicates all hormonal functioning and is a big factor in many chronic illnesses, especially for females.

The best water would be spring water from the mountains, and you'd still have to be careful about pollution. There are some websites where you can find out the closest place with tested spring water, which you can go collect. It may be a mission to go every week or so, but taking into consideration how water plays such a big part in our body, this effort seems to be a small one.

If you don't have access to spring water it's still better to get a good water filter. If installing a filter for your entire household is too much, start by filtering your drinking water first. There are many filters available out there and its very important to research them well to find out how effective they are.

NON – TOXIC COOKWARE

This was one of my biggest and unexpected changes. I was sitting on my sofa, basically covered with holistic books, noticing that one after another had a chapter about toxic cookware. TEFLON and any other non-sticky substances our cookware is covered with are highly toxic! According to the Environmental Working Group, when we heat a Teflon pan and temperatures exceed the point where the coating breaks apart, toxins are emitted through particles and gases. Also, during cooking, if Teflon pans are scratched, small amounts of plastic (dioxins!) and aluminum are stuck to our food and consumed by us!

After reading another chapter on non-toxic cookware in yet another book, I put it down and rushed to my kitchen. I opened my cupboard and after about forty-five minutes of taking inventory, I was left with one non-toxic cooking pot! All of my pans (except the one I left) were a non-stick style. The next day I went pan shopping and swapped out all aluminum, Teflon, copper and lead-glazed cookware for stainless steel, glass, cast, and Pyrex. I've found stainless steel and glass to be the best and the cheapest.

You don't have to make such a radical move as I did and chuck all your cooking pans in one go. You can purchase one by one until you have your dream set. The most important thing is having the awareness and the willingness to change. Also, please remember that cooking pans can last for a very long time if looked after properly. It may be an unexpected expense, but it's well worth it for the sake of your health.

I also made changes to my food storage containers. The majority of the ones I used to own were plastic. Because of dioxins, I changed them all for glass. Many shops these days are selling them quite cheap. I didn't get all of them at once. I changed the size I use the most and slowly built the set I wanted.

Look around your kitchen. Maybe there are other things you would like to change from plastic to glass? Consider a trip to vintage or second-hand markets and shops. I found so many beautiful jars to store my dry food and herbs in for very little money.

COSMETICS & CHEMICALS

Our skin is our biggest organ, and anything you are putting on it — (shampoo, body wash liquid, body cream, perfume, face cream, nail polish, nail varnish, makeup, makeup remover... the list goes on!) gets absorbed. Every day your body is absorbing the chemicals in your products. They are going directly into your system.

Unfortunately, the majority of cosmetics contain extremely harmful ingredients! Today, cosmetic manufacturers have no legal obligations to go through a pre-market approval process of their product before selling them in stores, and regulators do not assess the safety and effectiveness of the claims on the products. Instead, people and doctors are asked to report any health problems to the FDA's database. You would hope that in such an advanced world there would be much more protection for the consumer, but there isn't!

Below are some of the chemicals I came across when I started paying attention to and clearing out my cosmetics collection. Remember when I said to you I think endometriosis is just a side effect of something bigger, and toxicity of our environment and body have a huge impact on chronic illnesses? These are some of those environmental toxins. Hence, 'clearing' your environment is so important, especially what goes on your skin.

Chemicals:

- **1,4 Dioxane** — Not listed on ingredient labels, 1,4-dioxane is a contaminant linked to cancer found in products that create suds, such as shampoo and liquid soap.
- **Acrylates** — Acrylates (ethyl acrylate, ethyl methacrylate, and methyl methacrylate) are ingredients found in artificial nail products. They are linked to cancer, organ toxicity, and neurological issues.
- **Benzophenone** — A chemical linked to cancer, benzophenone is used in cosmetics such as lip balm and nail polish to protect the products from UV light.
- **Butylated Compounds**—Butylated hydroxyanisole (BHA) and butylated hydroxytoluene (BHT) are used as preservatives in a variety of personal care

products. Both of these chemicals are also used as preservatives in foods and cosmetics. These chemicals are linked to several health concerns including endocrine disruption and organ-system toxicity. They are found in lip products, hair products, makeup, sunscreen, antiperspirant/deodorant, fragrance, creams.

- **Carbon Black** — Carbon black is a dark black powder used as a pigment in cosmetics such as eyeliner, mascara, and lipstick that has been linked to increased incidents of cancer.

- **Coal Tar** — This is found in shampoos and scalp treatments, soaps, hair dyes, and lotions. It is linked to cancer and organ toxicity.

- **Fluoride** — A by-product of copper, aluminum and iron manufacturing. Fluoride helps the brain absorb aluminum, a substance that has been found in most of the brains of Alzheimer patients. Fluoride is linked with hip fractures as well as musculoskeletal and nervous system damage, which leads to limited joint mobility, ligament calcification, muscular degeneration, and neurological deficits. It's also linked to cancer.

- **p-Phenylenediamine (PPD)** — A chemical used in hair dye that is linked to lung and kidney problems and bladder cancer.

That's only a 'few' of the harmful chemicals, but for me, even this short list gave me solid motivation to have a closer look at what I put on my skin. It all sounds scary, I know! But I'm sharing this because I know what you are going through and I'm here to help as much I can. As I've said before, I invite you to do your own research after every chapter because I want you to learn how to develop ownership over your health. No book, guru, teacher, doctor or another endo woman can tell you how to treat your body. I can only share my story and what I discovered in five years of researching and taking care of my body. You are not alone in this journey.

My rule is simple — I put on my body only things that I'm prepared to eat!

So how did I become more careful about cosmetics? First, I changed the products I use every day, like shampoo, body gel, and intimate hygienic gel. I replaced them for paraben free, organic products that use natural essential oils for fragrance. I was able to find these at the local health store. There are many products out there, and some that you will be able to try before purchasing if you ask for a sample. I also reduced the variety of products I use. Now, I only use shampoo and intimate hygienic gel, which I also use on my body and face while showering.

Those products are super delicate and very good for any skin type.

I have many friends who worry that using natural products will make their hair or skin worse. I tell them to be patient. Many of your skin and hair problems are because of using paraben-based cosmetics that damage your natural oils. Please trust the process. Your skin needs an adaptation period to come back to her natural vibrant state.

Another product I switched out was body lotion. This one was easy. I got a big tub of coconut oil, which I use as a body cream, make up removal, hair conditioner and of course, for cooking! During the winter, coconut oil suits me the best. During spring and summer I choose lighter oils. I make my own rose oil by mixing rosebuds and any base oil. You can find many nice body oil recipes out there.

For my makeup, I mainly use organic products. In general, I'm not wearing much makeup anymore, so this part was very easy for me. I also stopped coloring my hair because of the chemicals. I love my hair now! I wasn't able to grow it long before and now it's super thick, long and naturally wavy. Of course, if that's the thing you can't imagine removing from your beauty routine (dyeing your hair), there are many 'less toxic' products to dye your hair with that are based on natural herbal ingredients.

I also stopped wearing perfumes. Perfumes are full of chemicals that interfere with hormones and thyroid function. Instead, I use natural essential oils, which are just divine. I use the oils each day, depending on what scent I'm drawn towards. It's a lot of fun, it gives me a nice variation, I stay toxin free, and it's much cheaper than good perfume.

I also switched out my hygiene pads. I have some shocking news. Conventional tampons and pads are bleached white using chlorine dioxide, a chemical that is very toxic and dangerous. Also, the majority of tampons and pads contain perfumes too! We use these products so intimately, and all these chemicals get absorbed directly into our bodies. It's best to get unbleached, unscented, organic pads and tampons.

CHEMICALS IN OUR ENVIRONMENT

Unfortunately, our environment, both indoors and outdoors, is extremely polluted, and we can't always change it. What we can do is make small changes to improve our home environment. My catchphrase is, "There is always space to improve." I live by it and keep researching because I know there is always something new to learn.

BEDDING

The first thing I changed was my bed. I used to have a metal frame bed and I changed it for an untreated wooden frame. I also changed my mattress from foam to organic bamboo, wool, and cotton. I know, good quality mattresses are expensive, but if you think about it we spend 1/3 of our life in bed sleeping. So if you live ninety years, you'd be asleep for thirty of them!!! In my opinion, there is no 'too high' a price for a healthy, good quality mattress.

There are two reasons why I decided to change my bed. First, I discovered how toxic foam is. It's actually cancerous. The second reason was that the majority of our recovery happens in our sleep, so I wanted to make sure I gave my body the best recovery friendly environment that I possibly could. I also changed my pillows and duvet. The best ones are the ones stuffed with feather or wool. I invested in special pillows, which are also orthopedics, but that's not essential. I also changed out all my sheets for cotton and used a company called Samina, who specializes in holistic beds and bedding.

PAINT

My next step was painting my house with clay-based paint. I know this sounds excessive, and I don't want you to go crazy. You don't have to do this now, but in a year or two when it's time to refresh the walls in your house, it's worth it to have a look at healthy paint. In modern paints, there are many toxins that are very harmful to our health.

You may live in a rental accommodation or you don't have anyone to help you to repaint your house, and if this is you, don't worry. I'm sharing everything I changed because this book is about my journey, and I want to write everything hoping there will be at least one thing you will choose to improve your health. Maybe paint is one of them and maybe it's not.

PLANTS

I also invested in indoor plants. I never had any before this and it wasn't because I didn't like them. In fact, I love them. It just wasn't my priority to have them before until I discovered the benefits: clean air and improved mood! Some plants have amazing capabilities to clean out the air in a home. I invite you to take a little trip to your local garden center and speak to somebody who can advise you on what sort of plants to get. It all depends on how sunny or shady your place is. Today, I have between fifteen and twenty plants and I can't imagine my house without them. I have four in my bedroom and

I love looking at them. Not only do they clean the air but also they improve my mental state, which is so important for recovery!

CANDLES

Before endometriosis, I was a huge fan of candles. I had many of them, some scented, some for ambiance. You should have seen how quickly I collected and got rid of them when I found out what was in them. Most candles are made from paraffin, a petroleum by-product. To create paraffin, petroleum waste is chemically bleached, deodorized and made into a wax. When a candle is burned, it releases toxins: acetone, benzene, and toluene, which are known carcinogens. These are the same chemicals found in diesel fuel emissions! For me I didn't have to look for more research — this was enough!

Today, if I really want to enjoy a candle, I go for an organic, vegetable wax one infused with essential oils. I also have two diffusers at home for essential oils. I mix a couple of drops of essential oil with water and I let my diffuser do the job. Essential oils don't just smell good. They can also help to ease pain and aid sleep. I also use dry herbs as an aromatic trick for my house. Usually, I dry some oregano and thyme, tie it with a thin string and then burn it when I feel I need some aromatherapy.

CLEANING PRODUCTS

These were also some of the first things I changed in my house as well. I got rid of conventional cleaning and laundry products and I swapped them for healthier options. To my surprise, when I started experimenting with a variety of healthy cleaning products out there, I discovered baking soda and apple cider vinegar worked wonders, and are much cheaper than regular toxic bleach or bathroom spray! If you can't be bothered to mix soda and vinegar into a paste, you can choose 'healthier' options found at regular supermarkets.

CLOTHING

I also took a good look at my wardrobe and kept only clothes made of natural materials. With a couple of trips to a vintage shop, I'm sure you'll be able to find some lovely things to wear. If you are not planning on giving up your favorite polyester jumpers and dresses, that's totally fine. I invite you to at least think about your underwear and make sure they are breathable cotton ones.

RED LIGHT THERAPY

My red light lamp is a little gold nugget for me! My nutritionist had proposed that I get a red light lamp and start using it straight after my second surgery. To this day I can't believe how much wonder this little red thing has done for me.

Red light therapy is used in many ways. Red light produces a biochemical effect in cells that strengthens the mitochondria. Sounds a bit fancy — I know. Simply said, the red light helps to create more energy inside your cells, and with more energy, cells can function more efficiently and heal your body faster.

The main benefit of Red light therapy is its ability to repair tissue and wound health. That was the main reason why I invested in and used it religiously. I saw the results very quickly. You don't have to go through surgery to start using a red light. If you suffer from endometriosis, you have many wounds and scar tissue inside that need repairing and healing.

Red light therapy also helps with pains from stiff joints and muscles. Every endo girl and woman knows how endometriosis can create spasms in our muscles and pains in joints. The red light helps fight inflammation!

I used my lamp every day for 10–15 minutes for the first year after surgery. Today, I use the light every other day on my face and on my abdomen. I'm very careful during my period days. I don't have enough knowledge on using red light during menstruation, and twice have come across some research that wasn't promoting it, so for now, I hold off on using it when I'm bleeding. I keep my mind open and research a lot, so I invite you to do the same to make sure you are taking ownership of your body and endometriosis.

CANNABIDIOL OIL

"CBD Is The Best Anti-Inflammatory, Anti-Cancer, Anti-Anxiety Superfood You're Not Eating."

—Mind, Body, Green

There's still quite a lot of controversy around this oil, and it's a shame because the benefits are endless. In many countries, cannabidiol oil is still illegal. That's because it's produced from the cannabis plant, which is classified as a drug.

Using cannabis oils is often misinterpreted as drug consumption. The cannabis plant has so many beautiful components that don't involve THC, its psychoactive component. Cannabidiol oil has no significant psychoactive components. There could be traces of THC present because of the way oil is made, but it won't affect your state of mind, it won't make you an addict, and it won't even show up in a blood test. During the production of cannabidiol oil, they remove the psychoactive parts of the plant. There are also plants specially grown for cannabidiol oil that have very high CBD and low THC components.

To understand more about cannabidiol oil's benefits and the process of how it is produced, let's have a look at the cannabis plant itself:

- **THCA** — A non-psychoactive 'ingredient' found in a raw cannabis plant. While left to dry, THCA converts to THC. THCA offers an anti-spasmodic effect and anti-insomnia effect.
- **THC** — That's the main psychoactive component of the cannabis plant. It can create euphoria and a deeper sense of presence. Apart from that, THC also stimulates appetite by triggering receptors in your body to release hunger hormones. THC has anti-inflammatory properties and can help with conditions like depression, Alzheimer's disease, Parkinson's, stroke, and cancer.
- **CBDA** — Trichomes of the raw plant. CBDA has anti-nausea and anti-cancer properties. Known as cannabidiol, when heated, breaks down from

an acid form into CBD. The process of CBDA becoming CBD is called decarboxylation. CBDA has anti-nausea and anti-cancer properties.

- **CBD** — This has NO psychoactive properties. Recently, it's become very popular as more studies prove it has amazing healing and curing properties. What makes CBD more attractive to consumers and patients is that it doesn't have psychoactive effects. It also carries a significant anti-inflammatory component, which decreases bone re-absorption and cancer cell proliferation. On top of that, CBD oil has the potential to relieve stress, improves mood, relieve chronic and acute pain, alleviate skin irritation and itching, reduce nausea and vomiting, improve sleep, and reduce joint pain and inflammation.
- **CBC** — This also has NO psychoactive properties. Instead, it has antiviral and anti–inflammatory properties and is used in treating acne. It's also been shown to inhibit tumors and fight cancer.

Based on all that, you have to admit, the cannabis plant is pretty cool! I hardly use the word cool, but seriously, I feel there is a little applause needed for Mother Earth to have created such an amazing plant medicine! Don't you think?

Before you run to the local health store or look online for products, let me share a few things that will make it easier for you to get the right oil. First of all, cannabidiol oil is not cheap, and when you are looking for one to invest in, please don't look for the cheapest one! I know many people who tried to save a buck and came back to me saying it didn't work. When I asked where they got their oil from and what they paid, I knew exactly what the problem was!

To grow an organic cannabis plant, and then make carefully curated oil that retains all its healing properties takes time and money. Cannabidiol oil is not a cheap business but there are many companies cutting corners and selling their products for less to exploit the market of increased interest.

SO, make sure you are buying from a good supplier. The best ones are in the USA and can ship to pretty much everywhere in the world. Before ordering, make sure you check the percentage of CBD allowed in your country. In the UK, for example, the legal percentage is 1200, but in Brazil, it's 5600! To be fair, this can't be checked during transport, so if you get your hands on good CBD oil with a high percentage, it's up to you to take the risk! The company that I use is called Elixinol. I trust them the most because when I was new and looking for the right oil for me, they were very informative.

I know in some countries, only a doctor can give you a prescription for cannabidiol oil. Make sure you get one. Doctors may be not so happy and try to get you a chemical painkiller instead because they make more money out of it, but be persistent. Also, make sure you ask many questions at the pharmacy and check the company to ensure quality control.

Overall, it's an amazing natural product with plenty of research-supported benefits. It's also safe for animals! I give the oil to my dogs Mia and Max. They are both elderly dogs and it helps them with joint pain. CBD oil has been a lifesaver for me, and I take it every day, even when I don't experience pains.

Happy CBD hunting!

HAIR TEST ANALYSIS

I did my hair test six months before my main surgery. Basically, what a hair test analysis does is take a sample of hair from your head or pubic region and analyze the minerals in your body to tell you where you're out of balance. It can detect pretty much anything, including toxic metals.

Mine was a complicated case again! It took me over two years just to get rid of copper and mercury. I'm also a big believer that excessive copper has a significant impact on endometriosis. To this day, I'm on a supplement specific to my issues and feel a huge difference.

If you want a deep dive on this, it's best to find a clinic that specializes in this type of treatment. Have a look around where you live for a hair analysis clinic. I definitely would recommend having your hair test done.

THYROID AND ADRENAL GLAND TESTS

These two glands play a huge role in endometriosis. The resulting inflammation present in endometriosis leads to the destruction of thyroid cells, causing the thyroid gland to become underactive! The thyroid and adrenal glands are a team, so what happens with one intimately affects the other.

On top of the physical impact that endometriosis has on both glands, there's of course the mental impact. Endometriosis can create constant stress from the chronic pain, lack of support and understanding, feelings of helplessness, and so on. All of those mental symptoms have an impact on the adrenal glands and thyroid.

It's a cycle that is very difficult to break because an underactive thyroid and adrenal gland fatigue can add to feelings of depression. It's a very scary and overwhelming chain reaction. That's why on top of thyroid and adrenal glands tests, I would suggest you also have a brain chemistry test done. It's not the cheapest, but it will show you your levels of brain chemicals and give you more information on how you can take back control of your moods.

When my test showed I had an underactive thyroid and struggling adrenals, it was only confirmation of what I knew already. At the time, I already had an amazing nutritionist who had me on a six-month program that was working towards cleaning my body and supporting my glands. I went on a special diet, heavy in vegetables, good fats, and protein. With commitment, I was able to regulate and restore the functioning of my glands. Now, I still have tests done on a regular base for my thyroid and adrenal glands in order to stay on top of my health.

List of thyroid friendly foods:

- **Foods high in Iodine** — Seaweed
- **Foods high in Selenium** — Brazil nuts, sardines, beef, turkey and chicken
- **Foods rich in Pectins** — Apples, pears, and citrus fruits
- **Foods high in Zinc** — Pumpkin seeds, crab, lobster, legumes, nuts, and sunflower seeds
- **Foods rich in Vitamin D** — Oranges and sardines
- **Foods high in Fiber** — Beans and legumes

- **Foods high in Omega-3 fatty acids** — Sardines, salmon, walnuts and flax seeds

GREEN MAGIC POWDER & SUPPLEMENTS

Our body is in constant inflammation mode so in my daily practice I make sure I get all the best food, water, minerals, and supplements. Here is my list of the supplements and herbal mixes that I use daily:

- **Green Magic Powder** — It comes in a powder and contains a mix of beautiful superfood greens listed below:
- **Spirulina**, which has 25 times more carotene than carrots, twice the B-12 content of liver, is high in iron, and contains more antioxidants than regular superfoods.
- **Chlorella**, which is the richest food source of chlorophyll, and contains beta-carotene, helps normalize digestion and bowel function (especially helpful for endo women and girls who have recto endometriosis!), strengthens the immune system, stimulates anti-cancer activity, repairs and grows tissue, and is high in protein.
- **Barley and Wheat Grass**, which are high in chlorophyll and natural potassium, help to

remove toxins, purify and cleanse the blood, are high in iron, help to improve skin color and tone, and are a rich source of vitamins, minerals and enzymes.

- **Icelandic Kelp**, which contains naturally occurring lithium, minerals, natural Iodine, and is rich in protein and vitamins B. (Just a small but very important note from me. Please make sure when you buy Kelp you check where is it from. Kelp is amazing as a rich source of minerals BUT it is like a sponge and if it's collected from polluted waters you will get kelp that's overloaded with toxins, so have that in mind while buying).

You can buy all of your greens in a mix, just like mine, or individually.

Another supplement that I use on a regular base is an herbal mix for the liver called Liver Chi by New Spirit Naturals. It is a complex mix of mushrooms like Reishi, Maitake, and Shitake, which have massive healing properties. Liver Chi protects and restores the function of the liver and balances out the immune system. It also detoxifies your liver and protects it from damage associated with inflammation, infection and autoimmunity problems.

Another supplement I use is called YES PEO oils. It's a mixture of oils that play a role in fighting inflammation in your body. I take them in capsules. If you can't get a hold of the pre-made mix, you can buy a separate bottle of each oil, make a mix of your own that you store in a dark empty bottle, and take a tablespoon daily orally.

These oils are: Flax oil, Pumpkin oil, high linoleic Sunflower oil, Evening Primrose oil, and Extra Virgin Coconut oil.

I also use turmeric paste, which I call Golden Paste! Turmeric is a very powerful antioxidant with anti-inflammatory properties. I mix either grated fresh turmeric root or turmeric powder with heated coconut oil and some black pepper. I mix all these ingredients until I get a nice thick paste, and eat a spoonful a day. Turmeric also improves brain function, lowers the risk of getting brain disease, lowers the risk of getting heart disease, aids in cancer prevention, helps to prevent and treat Alzheimer's disease, and helps with joint stiffness. As you can see, it works magic!

I also try to drink two herbal teas daily. The best are the loose dry herbs instead of tea bags. Marigold, fennel, and ginger are some examples that I enjoy and that help with easing endo symptoms.

There will be occasions where I will take something extra just to test it. Basically, I will try anything that might help to fight inflammation. There are also days where I don't take anything. I try to be systematic about my supplements but I'm not obsessive. If I forget one day, I don't stress about it!

SOME THOUGHTS ON ESSENTIAL OILS

"I believe that for every illness or ailment known to man, God has a plant out here that will heal it. We just need to keep discovering the properties for natural healing."

—Vannoy Gentles Fite

In most ancient cultures, people believed plants were magical. For thousands of years, herbs were used for medicine, healing and rituals. Modern medicine has now drifted towards chemical and symptom treatment instead of addressing the root causes of illnesses.

I think plant oils are bad ass. The benefits of using them for your body, both externally and internally, are endless. They're pretty much magic. It's a shame that essential oils aren't used as much as they could be, and many underestimate their power.

Straight after my surgery, I started using two main oils religiously, Frankincense and Myrrh, and a few others on the side while healing. Here's why:

- **Frankincense oil** — It's an aromatic resin obtained from the Boswellia tree. Frankincense helps reduce stress, helps boost the immune system and prevent illnesses, has anti-inflammatory and anti-tumor effects, can kill harmful bacteria, heals the skin, improves memory, helps to balance hormones, and helps with digestion. This is just a SMALL list of its benefits. This oil is like a little miracle in a bottle!
- **Myrrh oil** — A resin obtained from a tree called Commiphora, common in Africa and the Middle East. Myrrh has antioxidant properties, is very supportive in the recovery of liver damage, has antibacterial and antifungal benefits, is anti-parasitic, helps to heal skin and wounds, and is also used for relaxation.
- **Lavender oil** — An amazing antioxidant that prevents and can even reverse diseases, supports brain functioning, improves moods, and helps with stress. It's also used in treatment for diabetics.
- **Oregano oil** — A natural alternative to antibiotics, it's an anti-bacterial that fights infections, fights candida, has anti-inflammatory properties, and helps with allergies.

Those are just only four of my favorite essential oils. My list is much, much longer and I could definitely write another big chapter about essential oils and how much they can benefit your life. Perhaps in another book!

An oil diffuser was one of my best investments. Usually, I have my favorite oils defusing for an entire day. Mixed with water, a couple of drops will last for hours.

As I mentioned, I also use essential oils as perfume. You can mix the ones you like together or buy a ready-made mix. Just make sure before you apply some of the oils on your skin you mix them with coconut oil. Some essential oils are very powerful and when not diluted, can irritate your skin if you are sensitive. While buying them just speak to your supplier and ask for more information regarding dilution.

FINAL THOUGHTS

I know all of this information at once might feel overwhelming, especially if you either think you may have endometriosis, have been diagnosed, already had surgery, or are taking care of somebody who is experiencing this illness, maybe a friend, family member or lover. Perhaps you read this book because you simply want a change in your life and you feel that you are ready to create space to improve your health. The thing to remember is that you don't have to apply all the changes in one go. You don't have to apply all of them at all, to be fair. It's your body and you have a choice to take whatever you need from this chapter and go at your own pace. It's important to take ownership of and understand your body and its needs. If you listen to it out of love, not fear, you will find answers — I promise!

CHAPTER SIX

I Am Not a Victim

"I am not a victim. No matter what I have been through, I'm still here. I have a history of victory."

—Steve Maraboli

I'm very surprised at how quickly I pulled it together and "got on with it" after receiving a doctor's confirmation of my diagnosis. I immediately began researching, studying, and preparing for all the potential future outcomes that endometriosis could bring to my life on top of what I was already being with. Experiencing a chronic illness like endometriosis can be very challenging. As I've mentioned, it comes with intense physical and mental pains that can leave women feeling helpless, wanting to give up, and victimized. I want you to know that I feel you, I understand you, and I hear you. I am one of you, and we are not victims.

My strategy was simple. I trusted that there was some beautiful meaning to it all. I knew this disease was calling me to take better care of myself and I understood it was 'given to me' for some higher purpose. At the time of writing this book, I now know the reason — to be a light to others struggling on this journey, to connect with you, support you in your own healing journey, and remind you that you are not alone. If I didn't believe in the power of this experience and all I have gone through, I wouldn't be able to write this book.

In order to start making meaning of all this, I had to decide to give up the idea that I was a victim of this illness. It was hard because even while I was so busy researching, looking for cures, visiting doctors, and experimenting, sometimes everything felt so overwhelming for me. Victim mentality crept in from time to time and it was a big stretch for me to understand, accept, and embrace endometriosis.

You may ask, "How is it even possible to accept an illness that took pretty much everything from you... exercise, ease of travel, pain-free periods, dancing, joyful sex, vitality, jobs, dreams, kids, normally functioning organs… the list goes on?"

Well, I started with gaining an understanding of endometriosis. I knew I had no choice but to get to know her since I would be living with this illness for a long time, possibly forever. I wanted to become best friends with her so that we could work together, not in resistance.

When I researched endo, I went in with the attitude that I was researching one of my favorite subjects, like actors, artists, or plays. I also started to talk about endometriosis like I was talking about a person. I trusted that she wasn't there to hurt me and that she came to me because there was a bigger underlying issue to address. I knew I could learn a lot from her.

From that point on, acceptance came very quickly. With acceptance came the understanding that I was not a victim, and I that didn't want to be called "a sick person." I didn't want this disempowering language around me. I became an empowered woman who took care and ownership of herself and her body. I stepped into some BIG work, and there's nothing to pity about that. Reflecting on this, my heart is full of love! In fact, it's bursting!

I know reading this might make some of you cringe, and maybe you think I'm making this up, or am disconnected, but I'm the most connected I've ever been. As much as it takes physical work in order to feel better, you also have to do the mental and spiritual work to sustain the benefits.

Don't think that I never have days where I just want to give up, where I don't want to be understanding of 'something' what took away so much for me. I have challenging days, but not many anymore, and if challenges arise, I ALLOW myself to feel angry, disappointed, and frustrated. BUT, I never give up. I never stop accepting. I never ask the question, "Why me?!" This question doesn't exist in my world anymore. There is no winning in victim mode.

If you don't feel or understand this now, that's fine. It will come. Acceptance will come and that sense of "I'm a victim" will go. The sooner the better, but don't punish yourself if you don't feel it just yet. Just gently practice feeling into it, feeling ALL your feelings and not making them mean anything in the moment. Maybe you were just diagnosed by a doctor, maybe you have diagnosed yourself, or maybe you already had surgeries. I don't know what place you're in right now, but I do know you are strong and that you are capable of getting to know and accept your situation. You are experiencing endometriosis, which means you are a warrior, and powerful warriors have the capacity for forgiveness and acceptance.

During my process of acceptance, I discovered how scared I was to say out loud, "I accept that I'm experiencing endometriosis." There was this fearful resistance. It was almost like I was scared that if I said it out loud people would dismiss my pain even further and question if what I was experiencing was real. It always felt like I had to convince people that I wasn't lying about my pains and symptoms. I had to always defend my condition in order to get the support I needed, so if I admitted that I was ok with experiencing this chronic illness, would people completely discredit my pain? People already doubted me, but I realized that in the grand scheme of things, this didn't matter.

You and I are here to take ownership of what's happening with our bodies, to put all our focus into self-support, and to thrive. We are not here to prove whether or not we feel well at any moment. That's not your objective, WOMAN. You are beyond that, beyond being a victim and doubting yourself. Know that I see you, and I love you.

And remember…

**It won't be easy. Important things
are never easy.**

CHAPTER SEVEN

Taking Ownership of your Own Health, Soul, and Body

It's scary to hear that you are sick. Trust me, I get it. It can be so overwhelming that many of us jump to the quickest fix the doctors propose. In doing so, we perhaps make a decision that actually goes against our body's needs, a decision that tackles a symptom but ignores what's at the root of our condition. Perhaps we wait for others to tell us what to do or decide our fate. In my darkest hours of pain, I was right there, begging for anything to just take it all away. But there was a still small voice I held onto, the one reminding me that there was a different way.

Don't get me wrong about the physical treatment of conditions. Modern medicine does miracles, and if I had an accident and I broke my leg, modern medicine can absolutely help "put me together" again and recover. When it comes to more internal illness though, I think modern medicine very quickly reaches for what I like to call "short cuts" and dismisses many variables and conditions that surround the problem.

I will talk about this more in another chapter, but for now, I will tell you very quickly what I believe had a big impact on my health. First of all, the way I consumed food as a child and the amount of toxicity in my food greatly impacted how I felt. Secondly, I have trauma stored in my body from my relationship with my father and from witnessing domestic violence. Self-love was not modeled for me either as a child, and I received little attention and acceptance for who I was, which led to negative self-talk. These are just SOME of the first things that come to mind. I could write an entire book on my traumatic experiences, but that's not the point. We are not here to play the victim; we are here to be warriors together and to find a way to cure our bodies and souls.

The good news is that your body wants to thrive, to be healthy and in service for you to explore and experience this thing called LIFE. Our job is to give back to it by taking care of what we eat, how we move, how we let stress affect us, what sort of environment we live in, what sort of relationships we have, and activities we're a part of.

When I was diagnosed, I was at a stage where I already knew a bit about holistic healthcare. I had read a good number of books and watched some eye-opening documentaries about health, mind, and body. I understood the connection between what we eat and how we feel. The most important realization for me was that modern medicine and the sustainable treatment of disease are often independent of each other.

If you're reading this book, well done. You are taking ownership and starting a beautiful journey of exploring and understanding your body even more. Your heart and mind are open to receive and accept that there are many ways to heal disease.

It took me a while to get from feeling like a victim of my circumstances to a warrior and a beacon of hope for others. You may ask, "How the fuck do I stay positive in times when I can't even get up from my bed?" Again, I understand – More than you can imagine! But you have two options: One is to stay in bed, hate your life, give up, and wait for a miracle,

OR you can research FROM YOUR BED, educate yourself, tune in with your body and BE a miracle!

I definitely don't always have things sorted out. I still have days full of fear and feelings of giving up! It's very hard to always be "good vibes only" when you experience chronic illness, but I try to tune back in with what I desire to manifest in my life…which is to CURE MYSELF! That's right! I wonder how many of you ALLOW YOURSELVES to say that loud?

It took me quite a long time to allow myself to think that, let alone say it out loud, or write it down.

Here's an exercise for you to play with.

Take out some paper and a pen and finish this sentence:

I'm not allowing myself to think I could cure myself because…

Please focus on all the stories and beliefs that come up for you.

Now I invite you to release those beliefs as you allow for possibilities by finishing this sentence:

I'm allowing myself to cure because…

Be spontaneous and free in your thoughts. Imagine without limitations!

Finally:

When I cure myself, how will my life be different? What will it look like?

Doing this exercise will help you bring deeper awareness to the stories that are running your mind. There is often SO much conditioning from loved ones and society that we take on as truth, when in fact, they're just stories, and we have the power to author and choose new ones. You'll most likely find that the limiting beliefs that came up are NOT absolute truths, so why not break them down and bring them to the light?

When I diagnosed myself, I went from doctor to doctor, telling them that there was something wrong and that I felt I had endometriosis. Guess what they told me? "No, it's not endo. You just have a heavy period that's all. You experience pain every day because it's in your head! Stop thinking about it, take painkillers, try this medication," and the list goes on. Finally, when I got formally diagnosed they told me there was no cure. The only solution would be to have a hysterectomy or force my body into early menopause with hormonal treatment. I was thirty-four years old at the time. "Take pills for the rest of your life and stop your periods," they said!

If I managed to question all of it, so can you! I won't promise you it will be an easy ride. It will be a very difficult journey, full of tears, doubts, and moments where you will want to give up. But it will also be very rewarding and uplifting. It will nurture strength and confidence in your being.

So I invite you to take OWNERSHIP of your body and mind and step up for yourself. I would go so far as to say it's the most difficult thing you will EVER do, taking your health into your own hands. That's pretty scary, right? There will be no one to blame for the mistakes that you might make, for your pain, for the time invested in yourself, for the illness to potentially progress first instead of healing. There will be only you and the disease. Only you to "blame."

But then I encourage you to ask: How do you understand "blame" as a word in this scenario? I invite you to start shifting from that word and swap it out for "ownership." Ownership implies CHOICE, and with choice comes power. You didn't have a say in what happened to you has a child, or what may show up in your future, but you DO have a choice in how you will respond.

To me, this word "ownership" was and still is like an internal guidance system for me, a GPS if you like. It guides me every single day when I prepare a meal, when I move my body, when I take my supplements, and when I do any routine that helps me to thrive while simultaneously experiencing illness. There is still pain that shows up, days that I spend in bed, but now I take these experiences as messages from my body telling me, "It's time for a bit of self-love."

All of this might sound overwhelming, like there is no way you can get this all under *complete* control. And guess what? You never will! That's the beauty of it. It's a relationship, not a dictatorship with your body, and this relationship thrives off of acceptance. What you *can* do instead of panicking and allowing yourself to become more and more overwhelmed is work your way through things that have built up over time and caused you this disease in the first place. As much as you are experiencing physical symptoms, your pain stems from traumas and old belief systems that were seeded within you as a child. This self-sabotage, resistance, and pain in your soul is deeply related to your physical symptoms and can be healed through awareness, acceptance, and love.

WHY AM I EXPERIENCING DISEASE?

In my opinion, it is very important that you understand that as a whole, you are made of both spirit (or energy as I like to call it), and a physical body. I invite you now to remember a situation when you experienced some degree of stress. Did you notice that it created any physical symptoms like nausea, headache, or fatigue? This is because our thoughts trigger emotions that carry frequencies, and these energetic frequencies affect our physical bodies. So when we experience a trauma, it creates thoughts, emotions, and memories that are stored in our bodies as energy, and if we don't learn how to clean up our energy, this suppression can create disease!

It's impossible to release years of stored trauma all in one go and you don't want to put yourself in a 'rat race' to heal yourself because that would create more stress! This is all a process that needs patience and time. But it begins with taking an honest assessment of the experiences in your past and present that are now contributing to your stress and illness.

My suggestion is to find a comfortable place, put some nice music on, maybe some essential oils if you can get a hold of some. You could invest in good quality paper or a journal for processing your healing. Make this release a ritual. Make it special. It's your first step towards healing.

When you're ready, center yourself with a couple deep breaths, and on a sheet of paper, write down a couple of things that you think could be having an effect on the illness you are experiencing right now. These could be traumas you've experienced in your childhood, stressors that are going on today, or self-talk that feels unkind. Please make sure you take your time. There is no rush. This process can be painful and requires a lot of patience and commitment. Trust the process. It's all worth it.

At the end of this book, I will share a list of books that have helped me go deeper in my healing journey. I would recommend checking out at least a couple of books from the list. Healing is very personal, and everybody heals differently, which is why it's so important to invest time, do research, and review different sources to find what serves us best.

CHAPTER EIGHT

Forgiveness & Letting Go

I grew up in a very dysfunctional family unit with a father struggling with alcoholism and a mother who was depressed and co-dependent. They used the best tools they had to show us love and security in their own way. I know these traits were passed on from generation to generation. Unfortunately, before I had enough tools to understand why my parents (or anyone for that matter) behaved the way they did, I made up a story that I was a victim. As you can imagine, this was extremely toxic for my soul and body.

Often I'd be sitting on the sofa, driving my car, or walking my dog while simultaneously having aggressive, hypothetical conversations in my head with people who had hurt me. I would imagine hurting them back with my words and would think in so much detail and focus that these conversations could go on forever. In these moments, my body would tighten, my jaw would clench, there'd be heaviness in my chest, and I'd feel intense waves of restless and aggressive energy. I'd struggle to sleep, and when I did, I'd wake up with anxiety and a shaking in my chest.

Reflecting on it now, it was nuts. Every time we think about some sort of trauma or negativity from the past, our body reacts EXACTLY the way it would as if the situation was happening in the NOW moment. So in other words, when you think about a bad break up, an argument with a friend, an accident, a rape, or physical abuse over and over again, each time you are reliving and deepening the pain of this story. Your body doesn't have the ability to understand that it's only a memory. Your body and soul think this PAST you are thinking about is happening now in this REALITY again and again. There is no difference between what you experience for real and what you imagine.

Try out this exercise to see what I mean:

Lemon visualization

This exercise is quite popular and very easy. Close your eyes and imagine you are eating a lemon. Imagine the bitter taste and the juicy texture. You will notice that as you reflect on this, your mouth waters!

It's a simple but powerful example of how visualizations and thoughts lead to emotions and physical reactions in your body.

That's why it's so important to learn how to forgive and let go. First, you have to decide that you are willing to release your attachment to the pain. This can only be done if you are really willing and committed to healing. Then comes a commitment to love and acceptance, which were my most important tools for forgiveness. These were birthed from an understanding that everyone is doing the best they can do in the moment with the tools they have.

For me, forgiveness and letting go were the most amazing things I have done for my body and soul. When I accepted that I couldn't change other people and certain situations, my whole vibe changed. I experienced less digestive issues, less pain, and better moods.

Now I get that this is a process. You see, I was addicted to negative thinking so much that I thought without those memories, I would lose my identity. It sounds crazy but that's what I believed! Also, I was actually scared to be happy. I didn't think I deserved to be loved, to feel joy, to just be. I thought pain was the best outfit I had, and I stuck to this mask for a very long time.

There were a few questions I came across in my journey that began to put things in perspective for me. One was, "What is the benefit of staying in victim mode and creating drama?" Well, I realized that I got attention. People would validate me and I felt seen and accepted in my pain when I led with that story. But then I had to sit down with myself and get really clear on, "What's the cost of believing this identity?" Well, I was always sourcing validation from somewhere else, so my self-worth and happiness were dependent on how others saw me.

So I started playing with the idea that I am always enough and that I don't need validation from other people. I also started hanging around people who refused to see me as a victim. The more I released the victim story, the more these people just came into my life! I was attracting new connections and support from an empowered place.

I'm still in the process of forgiveness and I don't think there will ever be a finishing line, because we're always evolving and growing. We have a past and we're going to have a future. There will be always something new to heal, to forgive and let go, but as soon as you commit to this process, each 'bad event' will be easier to forgive and move on from.

When I started my process, I wanted to talk to everyone who had hurt me, and attempt to "clear the air." Quickly, I discovered that I have zero control on other people's perceptions. So instead of reaching out to every single person and burning up my energy, I focused on the inner work of letting go.

This was the hardest part for me because I didn't understand why people couldn't just change. I was still holding onto a hope that I could help them see the world through my eyes. So I also had to 'let go' of this idea and this desire to control others.

Forgiveness and acceptance are like besties. In my opinion, they come as a pair, and releasing this story around controlling others helped me to learn a few things about forgiveness. At first, I thought it would be easier to accept than to forgive. But as I started to accept and move from a space of Love rather than fear, forgiveness came with ease.

There are many activities on forgiveness and letting go, and I invite you to explore the literature on these processes. You can practice through meditations, journaling, and guided videos of movement. Everybody is different and perhaps will need different tools and techniques. There is no set recipe on how to do it, but a willingness to try different ways to heal is key.

Healing is not easy, but it will empower you in ways you can't imagine. Trust me. You will become a warrior, your own best friend and protector, and you will have much more compassion for others.

This journey was transformational for me, and it continues to be! It was a simple yet big puzzle piece to the healing of many of my conditions and wellbeing in general. Now it has a huge impact on how I deal with people, situations, physical pain and my mood. I can see my patterns of behavior and physical pains much more clearly. Sometimes I'm amazed that I managed to ignore the truth of my body and mind for so long!

One of my coaches asked me a question. "What does self-love means to you?"

My answer was: A willingness to heal!

CHAPTER NINE

Tapping Into My Womanhood

"What a beautiful woman. She moved with grace, she was entirely feminine, and yet, she possessed incredible inner strength. She's a survivor."

—Jan Moran

Since I was born, I identified as a girl, and then when I grew up, as a woman. There were a lot of do's and don'ts imposed upon me within this cis gendered identity. There was a lot of conditioning about my sex and looking back I can remember glimpses of sentences, events, words and conversations that defined how I understood myself by other people's standards. Most of the beliefs I took on were limiting and unloving.

I see endometriosis as a huge blessing because it gave me the opportunity to explore the subject of womanhood and question everything I had been taught. To start, I learned so much more about my anatomy, and it was shocking to realize how little I knew about my own womb, ovaries and fallopian tubes. I learned about my ovulation and the step-by-step process of my cycle, and I learned that it's OK to talk about my period. I learned more about my sexuality and how dynamic and pain-free sex could be. I learned the language of my body so we could communicate better. I discovered what serves my body, what does not, and that my body wants to serve me! I learned that my body could often heal on its own with little help from me. I learned to accept my curves more then I used to, and how to speak to my own womb. I learned how to stand up for myself, to take ownership of my own body and mind and stand in my feminine power. I also learned how to ask better questions and stand up for other women. I learned that it's ok to be open with my sexual partners and ask for more. I learned to talk about my physical and mental pain from a place of love, not victimhood. I learned to accept the fact that I'm experiencing chronic illness. I learned how to receive, and that I'm worthy of receiving. And finally, I realized that endometriosis has chosen me to share my journey with each of you in order to bring hope and healing.

This list is long, but I feel I only touched surface. All of the blessings mentioned above helped me to tap into my womanhood. While I regret nothing now, I did have to climb over a huge wall to get to the place where I can see it all in this light. That wall was my old beliefs around what it meant to be a woman.

I grew up in a traditional family, where the woman was the one usually working full time to take care of the house, cook, watch the kids, clean, food shop, etc. There was pressure not only to keep things in order but to look good while doing it too. The expectation was also to give birth. It was clear that if we had a womb, we should be birthing babies, and if we weren't, something was wrong with us.

Through this rigid conditioning, I developed some limiting patterns. I became shy, scared and ashamed to talk about sex and my body the way I do today, and I never stood up for myself as a woman who didn't want to just cook, clean and raise kids. I struggled to embrace that I had a bigger purpose and could do whatever I wanted with my life.

As a result of endometriosis and the research I began to do on womanhood, I opened up and dissolved these old beliefs with each new understanding. With knowledge came softness and acceptance. It was like a chain reaction.

I have to be raw now and say that not all of the information I came across gave me great comfort initially. Some of it felt very uncomfortable and unclear. Lots of resistance would arise along with lots of questions. I see now that it was all for a reason. This was how it felt to break old patterns and release beliefs. It was uncomfortable before it got better.

Today, being a woman to me means that I can express what I feel and it doesn't mean I'm a "drama queen." I experience lightness and deep love around my sense of self. I take time to talk to my womb and the space around it. I'm more aware of how my hips move and the power they have! I touch my hair often and stroke my arms when I watch movies. I take time applying body lotion after having a shower. I write myself love letters and buy myself flowers. I know when to say no, and I'm working actively on my co-dependency issues. I celebrate and praise myself each time there is even a small win. I masturbate more and touch my body in a loving way.

I mentioned masturbation because in the past I associated this with something 'naughty' or negative. The process of experiencing my body through endometriosis helped me to open up about masturbation to others and mainly to myself. I allowed myself to learn more and it's been a beautiful process. All of those little yet big things had and still have a significant impact on how I'm tapping in with myself as a woman.

Taking care of and getting to know yourself again is the biggest gift you could ever give to you. Below are some exercises that I discovered during my journey or that were shared with me from other women. Please try to make some time for yourself during each day to engage in something that fills your cup. It can be short, long, simple or more dynamic, but prioritize something that reminds you that you are Love.

LIST OF SELF-CARE ACTIVITIES:

- Take a long bath with essential oils. You can even put on music and light some candles.
- In the morning when you wake up, stretch in your bed. Close your eyes and stroke your arms, belly, breasts, whatever you desire. The touch doesn't have to be sexual. Think about it as a loving stroke.
- Take yourself on a date. Book a table in the restaurant of your choice and go eat your favorite food.
- Buy yourself flowers.
- Buy yourself a cozy jumper or blanket.

- Watch your favorite movie.
- Curl your hair, put nice lipstick on, or wear your favorite outfit.
- Buy a book you've been wanting to read.
- Get yourself cashmere, or good quality wool bed socks.
- Take the day off and just spend it with yourself.
- Take yourself to the cinema.
- Write yourself a love letter – just like you would be writing from a lover to lover.
- Listen to a beautiful meditation.
- Put your favorite music on and have a dance.
- Plan a short trip/spa day.
- Watch an interesting documentary.
- Call your best friend or met him/her for healthy hot chocolate.
- Have a beautiful slow walk in the park.
- Make yourself an amazing meal.
- Cook yourself your favorite cake using healthy ingredients.

CHAPTER TEN

Sex & Relationships

Sex is so important to our health and pleasure. Among many other benefits, it can strengthen the immune system, improve bladder control, and lower blood pressure. However, for women with endometriosis, it can be a painful and even fearful experience at times! In both my own experience and those of the women I've interviewed, communicating the pain of sex with their partners can bring up a lot of resistance. Concerns I've both heard and felt are, "What if my partner leaves me or thinks I'm a bad lover?" Sometimes, women don't know differently ; they settle, uncomfortable sex is just the way it is.

    This fear of being abandoned was strong for me. Looking back, I think I chose less emotionally available men because it was easier for me to understand why they would walk away from a relationship with me. It made sense when my pain or discomfort was too much for them. It was also less risky for me to be hurt because I also held back emotionally. I never allowed myself to call in or experience deep love because I was too afraid that I would lose it. I thought that either way would be painful for me. There was no winning in this story.

My narrative was pretty ill-informed from the beginning though. I didn't know much about sex because no one spoke with me about it. All I knew was what I saw from little sneak peeks into pornography. This form of sex education was quite twisted.

The physical act was clear, but I never knew how to truly navigate my own pleasure. I didn't know that sex shouldn't be painful. I never questioned why the men I was with would orgasm and I would not. I never knew how to ask for more, or what I wanted. So I just existed with sex, no strong feelings, no real desires. Ninety-nine percent of the time I had sex just for the man's pleasure.

At the age of sixteen, I lost my virginity to my first boyfriend. Of course, the first time can often be painful in general, and many of you probably can relate. But my pain didn't get any easier, and I wasn't talking about it for fear that I'd lose or disappoint him.

Intercourse felt like a sharp stabbing with each push. Depending on the position, sometimes it was worse and sometimes it was less. Quite often I felt sick after, like I wanted to vomit. I would also get a bloated belly and have painful urination and bowel movements. Sometimes I would come down with a fever for a couple of hours, or my kidneys would hurt intensely. One time I almost fainted. It felt more like someone was beating me up than making love to me. Only once in a rare while would I have relatively pain-free intercourse.

When that man and I split, I met another man who was very understanding about my pains. He would ask me what I wanted and I felt safe telling him about what was going on in my body. We built an amazing connection and I felt understood and accepted. Sex was actually less painful. It was as close to love as I'd ever felt before, but we were young and ended up growing apart.

As time passed, I had a few more partners after him. Self-love wasn't on my radar yet so I was still outsourcing my self-worth from men and called in partners who were not as understanding. It felt like going back to square one. I thought I would never, ever put myself through the same experience, but back then I didn't know any better.

I'd so love to give my younger self a cuddle and have a heart to heart talk. I was just lost, as many of us are. There's so little education about male and female energy, about the nuances and dynamics of intimacy, and most importantly, about self-love.

Today, I believe all our power and transformation stems from self-love. If we don't commit to loving ourselves, then the majority of the things we do are done out of fear to avoid pain! I thought it was okay to share my body out of fear that I would disappoint my partner, and at the time, this potential of doing that felt more painful to me than the physical pain of sex.

It took me hitting rock bottom to realize that something had to change. I was thirty years old and had just lost somebody who I thought would be my partner for the rest of my life. Even that relationship wasn't great, but I was caught in a fairy-tale delusion that we'd be happily-ever-after. We'd gotten engaged and were planning our wedding when he came back home one evening and abruptly told me, 'It's over."

For the next six months, I lived in a black hole, crying, not eating, and feeling sorry for myself. The voice in my head was telling me I'd be alone for the rest of my life, that I wasn't worthy of love. On top of that, I kept bringing up memories of my ex telling me, "You are too demanding… you talk about what you feel too much… other mates have more easy going girlfriends." Between that and my own self beat-up, I felt depressed. My self-esteem was at ZERO.

From that space of darkness, I found myself desperately repeating my old patterns with yet another emotionally unavailable man, trying to feel a spark of love. I'm not sure I ever met anyone with so much anger and lack of self-love as this one. I dedicated all of my attention to him and got nothing in return. Usually, I got some validation, but this time, nothing. We fell pregnant and I had to terminate my pregnancy due to an "unexplained mass" in my uterus. Today I know that it was the build-up from endometriosis and adenomyosis, but for some reason, the doctor didn't speak to this then.

We had broken up and gotten back together many times already, but six months after this happened, we split for good. It was very painful to lose somebody again even though I knew that this man wasn't for me. My health issues became more visible and the pain was getting stronger and stronger around the clock.

To forget and recharge I decided to go to a yoga retreat in Sweden. There, I met a yoga teacher who very quickly became my lover for about three months. For the first time, I got to experience quality sex. It wasn't important for him to cum. He really wanted to give me maximum pleasure first. He never asked for anything, he was just giving. He was open to listening to what I needed and also gave me insight into understanding my body. He showed me there was another way to be with sex and that I could actually access deep pleasure in my body. With the freedom I felt to communicate about and honor my body came the freedom to relax, open up, and allow pleasure.

I don't regret any of the other men I shared my body with though. In fact, I thank the universe for bringing each of them into my life because I believe there was a lesson to learn with each one. I had to experience deep disconnection from my body in order to know and appreciate what powerful connection feels like. Nobody is to blame for my pain. Most of us are never taught how to build solid relationships or how to love ourselves before loving others.

Today, I have a totally different perception of my sexuality. It's more than just the physical act, but even the physical act has become more colorful. I'm not scared to stand up for myself and ask for what I need from a lover. As far as I'm concerned now, if a man wants to really connect with me, he needs to be open and willing to honor this.

Endometriosis and the experience of truly being honored by a man have created a "lover filter" for me. I smile as I write this because now I can tell who is really ready to show up for me. I connect now with more powerful and masculine man in bed. I may not have an intention to build relationships with them but I'm capable of having pleasurable and open sex.

I believe that each of you can also have deep conversations with your lover or partners about how you feel. I think this is such a beautiful way to connect and open up, not only for your relationship but more importantly, for yourself. It is very much an act of self-love, the initiation to another level of consciousness and understanding of your own body, and it will change your life. Trust your instincts and make sure you are taking care of your sexuality and yourself. If you desire further support in this area, I strongly encourage you to find a therapist or a mentor that can guide you through this process of advocating for your sexual needs. You don't have to go through this process alone.

I wish you lots of joy!

CHAPTER ELEVEN

Meditation

My relationship with meditation has changed over the past five years or so. I started to practice meditation in order to heal my depression, to understand more about how my mind worked, and to learn how to regulate my emotions. I was very experimental with different types of meditation and with my approach to how I put it into practice. Just like with everything, I never followed exact direction. I like to own every experience and explore as much I can.

In all honesty, back then I didn't take meditation too seriously. Yes, I could see some benefits, but I didn't have a sustainable internal drive, no divine need to sit and go within. I was driven more by what others were saying, like, "meditation is great for your wellbeing and you should try it." Hence, it wasn't regular or a priority.

Today, my approach to meditation has changed dramatically, as has its impact on my life. I'm not sure if the shift was a side effect of all the work I had done with healthy eating, mindful sex and trauma healing, but I actually started feeling like I "needed" to sit still and experience my body more. As I became more consistent with it, I started to feel this desire to just escape and be with myself. Maybe my body became more responsive and awake. It was like another level of awareness unlocked inside me. It was very natural, just like the urges of hunger we get when it's time to eat.

I don't believe that I have to be sitting still with my eyes closed to tune in. For me, meditation can be as simple as feeling my feet touching the ground while I'm walking, one foot after another. It's anytime I bring awareness to my body doing anything. In fact, that's how I started; feeling and focusing on simple touches, movements, breathing, and body functions. Now I choose where and what sort of meditation I will be doing depending on how I'm feeling that day. I'm more connected with my body and soul and have an understanding of what I need to do to make a space for that to happen.

As soon as I practiced this and was able to switch my focus from my mind to my body, I began to understand the real essence of meditation. It wasn't about clearing the mind, and yet it was. I still have thoughts, but they just pass by now and I don't hang onto them. I don't create stories and I'm able to focus on my intention, which is to feel, not think.

If I could give you a piece of advice, it would be to relax and don't become rigid around any meditation teaching. Sometimes when people start to explore different meditation practices, they put so much pressure on what it should look like. For example, some think they shouldn't have thoughts during meditation or that they should sit in a set position. I don't believe in should or shouldn't. My advice would be to do some research, experiment, explore what works for you, and relax around all that 'proper' stuff. Enjoy!

For You

I know I have told you before in previous chapters, but I want to tell you again. You are not alone, you are loved, you are supported, and you can get better. In this very moment, it may look or sound like there is no way out, but trust me, there is.

This book is for YOU. I see me in each of you. I see me in your experiences, and I see you in mine. I hope that by reading my book you have realized you are safe and supported in exploring your healing. I invite you to re-read it and make it your own journal. Please write on it, mark pages, sentences, or words. Note anything that stands out and brings you hope or healing.

I still remember the facial expression of my doctor when he told me, "You have a chronic illness." I can hear his voice distinctly and I remember the way my heart sank. It feels like it was yesterday. But since then, I've realized so much. When I look at my life, I see so much more than just a woman with chronic illness. You and I are much more then Endometriosis and Adenomyosis.

Please believe in yourself. Believe in the power of your body to heal. Believe in the power of healthy food, and the wisdom of your womb-space, your intuitive center. Believe in your ability to take ownership. Believe in your power as a Woman.

For you. For me. For her.

Recommended Reading

My Favourite Books:

Dear Lover by David Deida

A New Earth by Eckhart Tolle

The Power of Now by Eckhart Tolle

You Can Heal Your Life by Louise Hay

You are a Badass by Jen Sincero

A Return to Love by Marianne Williamson

Medical Medium by Anthony William

The War of Art by Steven Pressfield

The 9 Steps to Keep the Doctor Away by Dr Rashid Buttar

Conversations with God by Neale Donald Walsch

Endometriosis a New Zealand Guide by Andrea Molly

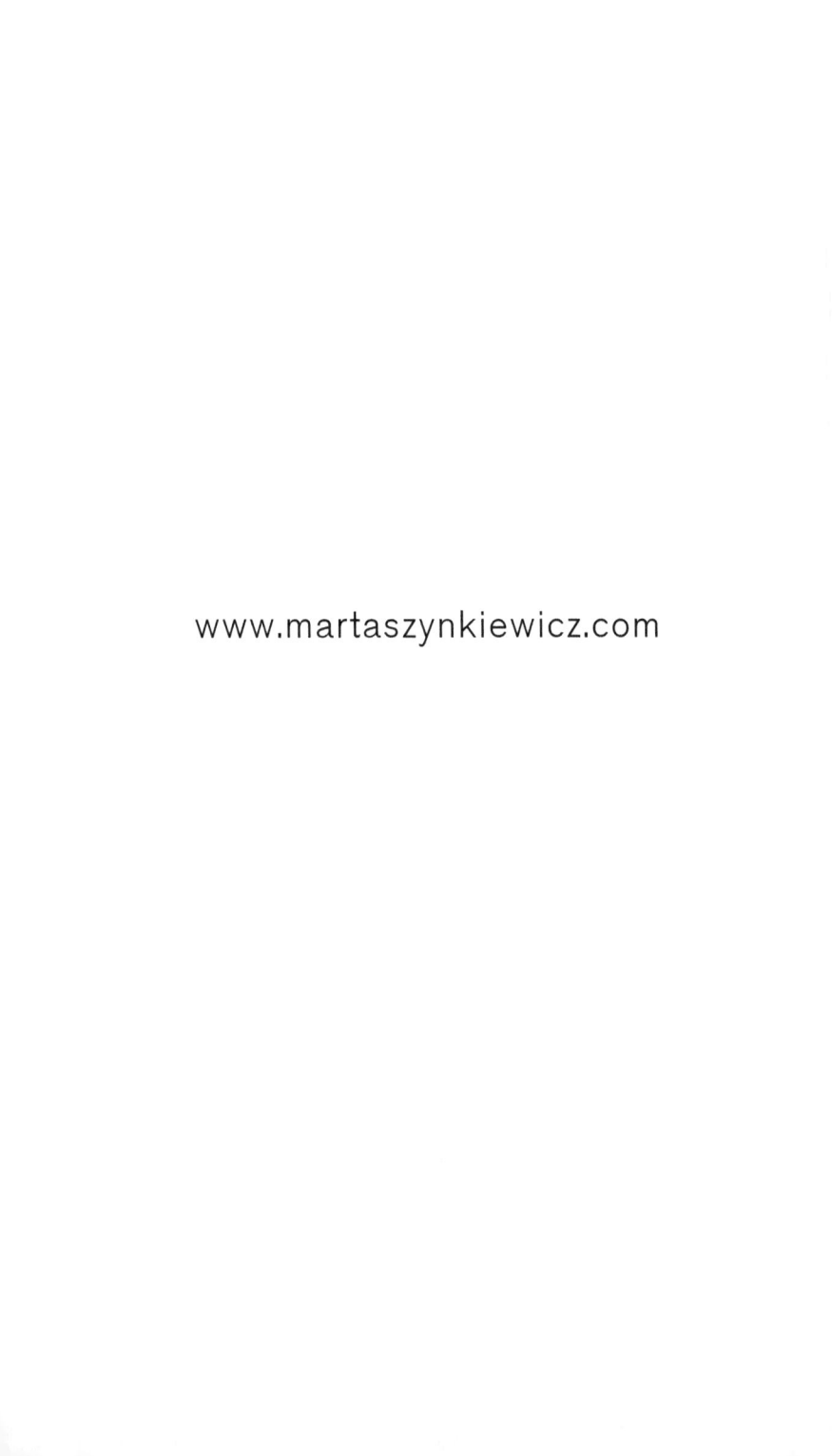
www.martaszynkiewicz.com